SINCE 1820

Founded in 1820, the **U.S.P. Convention** is responsible for establishing legally recognized drug quality standards in the United States—and for disseminating authoritative information for the use of medicines and related articles by health care professionals, patients and consumers. Over 1000 experts serve on USP Subcommittees and Advisory Panels and as *ad hoc* reviewers to ensure the accuracy and current relevance of USP standards and information.

THE

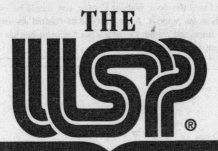

GUIDE TO
VITAMINS
& MINERALS

FIRST EDITION

By authority of U. S. PHARMACOPEIA

AVON BOOKS ◆ NEW YORK

The information on page v constitutes an extension of this copyright page.

AVON BOOKS
A division of
The Hearst Corporation
1350 Avenue of the Americas
New York, New York 10019

Copyright © 1996 by The United States Pharmacopeial Convention, Inc.
Published by arrangement with The United States Pharmacopeial Convention, Inc.
Library of Congress Catalog Card Number: 95-94914
ISBN: 0-380-78093-3

First Avon Books Printing: April 1996

AVON TRADEMARK REG. U.S. PAT. OFF. AND IN OTHER COUNTRIES, MARCA REGISTRADA, HECHO EN U.S.A.

Printed in the U.S.A.

RA   10 9 8 7 6 5 4 · 3 2

The inclusion in *The USP Guide to Vitamins and Minerals* of a monograph on any drug in respect to which patent or trademark rights may exist shall not be deemed, and is not intended as, a grant of, or authority to exercise, any right or privilege protected by such patent or trademark. All such rights and privileges are vested in the patent or trademark owner, and no other person may exercise the same without express permission, authority, or license secured from such patent or trademark owner.

The listing of selected brand names is intended only for ease of reference. The inclusion of a brand name does not mean the USP or Avon Books have any particular knowledge that the brand listed has properties different from other brands of the same drug, nor should it be interpreted as an endorsement by the USP or Avon Books. Similarly, the fact that a particular brand has not been included does not indicate that the product has been judged to be unsatisfactory or unacceptable.

NOTICE: The information about the drugs contained herein is general in nature and is intended to be used in consultation with your health care providers. It is not intended to replace specific instructions or directions or warnings given to you by your physician or other prescriber or accompanying a particular product. The information is selective and it is not claimed that it includes all known precautions, contraindications, effects, or interactions possibly related to the use of a drug. The information may differ from that contained in the product labeling which is required by law. The information is not sufficient to make an evaluation as to the risks and benefits of taking a particular drug in a particular case and is not medical advice for individual problems and should not alone be relied upon for these purposes. Since the inclusion or exclusion of particular information about a drug is judgmental in nature and since opinion as to drug usage may differ, you may wish to consult additional sources. Should you desire additional information or if you have any questions as to how this information may relate to you in particular, ask your doctor, nurse, pharmacist, or other health care provider.

Acknowledgments

The information in this book has been created primarily through the work of the USP Expert Advisory Panel on Nutrition and Electrolytes, chaired by Robert D. Lindeman, M.D. Ann Corken, DID Drug Information Specialist, served as staff liaison to the Panel and has been responsible for the development of the information. Harriet S. Nathanson (Editorial Associate) and Nancy Olins (Manager, Professional Affairs) also have contributed to the development of the information in this book.

For a complete listing of Advisory Panel and Headquarters Staff members, see the Contributors section, pages 269–321.

Contents

To the Reader   xv
  How to Use This Book   xv
  About USP   xvii
  About *USP DI*   xviii

Dietary Supplement Regulation/Quality   xxi
  Food and Drug Administration
    Regulation of Dietary Supplements   xxi
  Dietary Supplement Quality   xxii
  Vitamin and Mineral Product Quality
    Indicators   xxv

About Nutrition   xxvii
  Importance of Diet   xxvii
  Daily Recommended Intakes   xxxiii
  What Are Vitamins and Minerals
    and How Do They Work?   xxxiv

About Dietary Supplements   xli
  Fat-Soluble Versus Water-Soluble
    Vitamins   xli
  Are Natural Vitamins Better Than
    Synthetic Vitamins?   xlii
  Who Needs Vitamins and Minerals?   xliii
  Claims Made for Vitamins and
    Minerals   l
  Can I Take Too Much of a Vitamin
    or Mineral?   li

General Information About Use
    of Dietary Supplements   liii
  Proper Use of Your Dietary
    Supplement   liii
  Missed Dose   liii
  Storage of Your Dietary Supplement   liii
  Communicating with Your Health
    Care Professional   liv
  Considerations When Choosing a
    Dietary Supplement   liv
  Tips Against Tampering   lviii
  Unintentional Poisoning   lix

Dietary Supplement Monographs   1
  Ascorbic Acid (Vitamin C)   3
  Beta-Carotene   13
  Biotin   19
  Calcium Supplements   21
  Chromium Supplements   37
  Copper Supplements   41
  Enteral Nutrition Formulas   47
  Folic Acid (Vitamin B_9)   55
  Iron Supplements   61
  Magnesium Supplements   75
  Manganese Supplements   83
  Molybdenum Supplements   87
  Niacin (Vitamin B_3)   91
  Pantothenic Acid (Vitamin B_5)   97
  Phosphates   101
  Potassium Supplements   111
  Pyridoxine (Vitamin B_6)   125
  Riboflavin (Vitamin B_2)   131
  Selenium Supplements   135
  Sodium Fluoride   139
  Sodium Iodide (Vitamin B_1)   147

Contents

Thiamine 153
Vitamin A 157
Vitamin B$_{12}$ 167
Vitamin D and Related Compounds 173
Vitamin E 183
Vitamin K 191
Zinc Supplements 197
Glossary 203
Contributors 269
Index 323

List of Illustrations

Vitamin and Mineral Product
    Quality Indicators   xxv
Food Guide Pyramid   xxviii
The Food Label   xxx
How to Read a Supplement Label   lvii

TO THE READER

When purchasing a dietary supplement, whether over-the-counter (nonprescription) or with a doctor's prescription, you may have questions about its usefulness to you, the best way to take it, possible side effects, and precautions to take to avoid complications.

The USP Guide to Vitamins and Minerals contains information that may provide general answers to some of your questions as well as suggestions for the correct use of your dietary supplement.

How to Use This Book

The USP Guide to Vitamins and Minerals contains a section of general information about diet and dietary supplements, as well as detailed discussions of individual nutrients. Individual discussions (monographs) of these nutrients begin on page 3 and are arranged in alphabetical order by nutrient name. By looking in the Index, however, you can find either the brand name or the nutrient name of your dietary supplement and the page listing for the appropriate monograph. *You should read both the general information and the information specific to the nutrient or nutrients you are taking.*

Notice:

Depending on labeling and the particular law involved, a dietary supplement may be classified as a food or a drug. The information about the dietary supplements contained herein is general in nature and is intended to be used in consultation with your health care providers. It is not intended to replace specific instructions or directions or warnings given to you. The information is selective and it is not claimed that it includes all known precautions, contraindications, effects,

---

or interactions possibly related to the use of a dietary supplement. The information may differ from that contained in the product labeling, which is required by law for some products. The information is not sufficient to make an evaluation as to the risks and benefits of taking a particular dietary supplement in a particular case and is not medical advice for individual problems and should not alone be relied upon for these purposes. Since the inclusion or exclusion of particular information about a dietary supplement is judgmental in nature and since opinion as to dietary supplement usage may differ, you may wish to consult additional sources. Should you desire additional information or if you have any questions as to how this information may relate to you in particular, ask your health care professional.

Since previously unreported side effects, newly recognized precautions, or other new information for any given dietary supplement may come to light at any time, continuously updated information sources should be consulted as necessary.

There are many brands of dietary supplements on the market. The listing of selected brand names is intended only for ease of reference. The inclusion of a brand name does not mean the USPC has any particular knowledge that the brand listed has properties different from other brands of the same dietary supplement, nor should it be interpreted that that particular brand has been judged to be unsatisfactory or unacceptable.

The nutrient content definitions in this book have been simplified and are not necessarily consistent with those utilized for regulatory purposes.

If any of the information in this book causes you special concern, do not decide against taking any dietary supplement prescribed for you without first checking with your health care professional.

About USP

The information in this volume is prepared by the United States Pharmacopeia (USP), the organization that sets the official standards of strength, quality, purity, packaging, and labeling for drugs and nutritional supplements used in the United States.

The United States Pharmacopeia is an independent, not-for-profit corporation composed of delegates from the accredited colleges of medicine and pharmacy in the U.S.; state medical and pharmaceutical associations; many national associations concerned with medicines and dietary supplements, such as the American Medical Association, the American Nurses Association, the American Dental Association, the National Association of Retail Druggists, and the American Pharmaceutical Association; and various departments of the federal government, including the Food and Drug Administration. In addition, four members have been appointed by the Board of Trustees specifically to represent the public. USP was established 175 years ago, and is the only national body that represents the professions of both pharmacy and medicine.

The first convention came into being on January 1, 1820, and within the year published the first national drug formulary of the United States. The *U.S. Pharmacopeia* of 1820 contained 217 drug names, divided into two groups according to the level of general acceptance and usage.

When Congress passed the first major drug safety law in 1906, the standards recognized by that statute were those set forth in the *United States Pharmacopeia* and in the *National Formulary*. Today, the *USP* and *NF* continue to be the official U.S. compendia for standards for drugs and for the inactive ingredients in dosage forms. The *United States Pharmacopeia* is the world's oldest regularly revised national pharmacopeia and is generally accepted as being the most influential.

The work of the USP is carried out by the Committee of Revision. This committee of experts is elected by the members, with the 1990–1995 Committee consisting of 114 outstanding physicians, pharmacists, dentists, nurses, chemists, microbiologists, and other individuals particularly qualified to judge the merits of drugs and dietary supplements and the standards and information that should apply to them. Committee members serve without pay and are assisted by numerous advisory panels, other outside reviewers, and USP staff.

About *USP DI*

USP DI Volume I (Drug Information for the Health Care Professional) contains drug and dietary supplement use information in technical language for the physician, dentist, pharmacist, nurse, or other health care professional. Volume II (Advice for the Patient) is its lay language counterpart for use by consumers. Volume III provides information on approved drug products and legal requirements. The monthly *USP DI Update* keeps all volumes up-to-date with selected new entries and related information. Many health care professionals, institutions, and associations in the United States and Canada provide individual drug leaflets based on *Advice for the Patient*. Spanish translations for many medicines are also available.

USP DI was first published in 1980. It is continuously reviewed and revised and is intended for use by prescribers, dispensers, and consumers of medications and dietary supplements. The information is developed by the consensus of the USP Committee of Revision and its Advisory Panels and anyone, including users of medicines and dietary supplements, may contribute through review and comment on drafts of the monographs when they are published for comment in *USP DI Review*, a part of the monthly *USP DI Update*.

For further information about *USP DI* or to comment on how the information published in this volume might better meet your information needs, please contact:

> USP Division of Information Development
> 12601 Twinbrook Parkway
> Rockville, Maryland 20852
> (301) 816-8351

DIETARY SUPPLEMENT
REGULATION/QUALITY

Before 1993 there were few laws regulating the manufacture of dietary supplements or claims that companies could make about them. New legislation now regulates what manufacturers can claim about their dietary supplement products. In addition, guidelines for the quality of dietary supplements have also been developed.

Food and Drug Administration Regulation of Dietary Supplements

Dietary supplements are regulated as foods by the Food and Drug Administration (FDA). In October 1994, the United States Congress passed the Dietary Supplement Health and Education Act of 1994 to address issues that relate to the regulation of dietary supplements. Under this law, the FDA has the authority to regulate medicinal-use claims (e.g., cure for the common cold or prevents baldness) made by dietary supplement companies. However, companies are allowed to make general claims (e.g., strengthens the immune system) about their products without FDA approval. The FDA is also responsible for the safety of dietary supplements. In addition, the Act allows stores that sell dietary supplements to make scientific information available if it is presented in a balanced way.

Dietary Supplement Quality

The FDA does not establish standards for the quality of dietary supplements; however, they are in the process of establishing manufacturing guidelines for dietary supplements.

The United States Pharmacopeia (USP), which sets standards for drug products, recently established standards for vitamins and minerals. These standards include purity, potency, disintegration, dissolution, packaging, and labeling. Increasingly, these standards will enable consumers of dietary supplements to identify products whose quality can be trusted.

Dietary supplement manufacturers will be starting to alert consumers that their products meet the USP purity, potency, disintegration, and dissolution standards. As a result of official USP standards for dietary supplements, an increasing number of these products will feature "USP" on the label adjacent to the product's brand name. Be sure to look for this indication of product quality.

There are several key standards of quality that are important in making sure that dietary supplement tablets and capsules work in the body as expected. USP standards for the following indicators of quality are based on laboratory testing:

Disintegration—how fast a tablet or capsule breaks into small pieces so that its nutrient ingredients can dissolve. If a tablet or capsule does not break down within a certain amount of time, it may not dissolve and may pass through the body without its nutrient ingredients being absorbed.

Dissolution—how fast a vitamin or mineral substance dissolves in the intestinal tract once the tablet or capsule has disintegrated. If it does not dissolve, its nutrient ingredients cannot be absorbed into the body to do their work.

Strength—the amount of a specific vitamin or mineral substance in each tablet or capsule. To meet USP product quality standards, the amount present must be within a limited range of the amount declared on the label.

Purity—standards for purity provide limits for impurities that can result from a contamination or degradation of the product as a result of the process by which the product is produced, or of the manner in which it is stored.

Expiration Date—the date beyond which the nutrient ingredients in a properly stored bottle or package of supplements may no longer meet USP standards of purity, strength, and/or quality.

VITAMIN AND MINERAL PRODUCT QUALITY INDICATORS

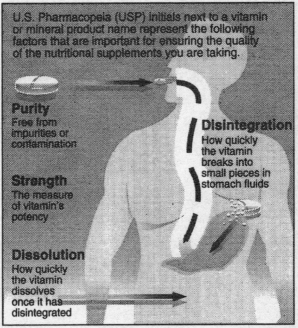

U.S. Pharmacopeia (USP) initials next to a vitamin or mineral product name represent the following factors that are important for ensuring the quality of the nutritional supplements you are taking.

Purity
Free from impurities or contamination

Strength
The measure of vitamin's potency

Dissolution
How quickly the vitamin dissolves once it has disintegrated

Disintegration
How quickly the vitamin breaks into small pieces in stomach fluids

Source: U.S. Pharmacopeia (USP), 1993.

ABOUT NUTRITION

Importance of Diet

For good health, eating a balanced and varied diet is important. Follow carefully any diet program your health care professional may recommend. For your specific dietary vitamin and/or mineral needs, ask your health care professional for a list of appropriate foods.

The Food Guide Pyramid

The Food Guide Pyramid is a standard you should use for a well-balanced diet. The Food Guide Pyramid (also called the Eating Right Pyramid) was developed by the Department of Health and Human Services and the U.S. Department of Agriculture. It represents a consensus of experts and is based on the scientific information currently available. The Pyramid has evolved from the previously used four basic food groups, and identifies the types of foods in each nutritional group. By using the eating plan in the Pyramid, you can make wise food choices to get the nutrients essential to good health.

Current research has found that those who eat more fruits, vegetables, and some grains and watch their intake of fats, cholesterol, and sodium have a lower incidence of certain diseases. For example, the National Cancer Institute recommends that eating 5 servings of fruits and vegetables a day may reduce your risk of developing cancer and cardiovascular disease. It is not known at what point in the life cycle this is important. It is also not known how much of a role other factors such as genetics, the environment, or obesity might play.

Note that you do not have to eliminate totally foods that are high in fats, cholesterol, and sodium. It is your average intake of these items over a few days, not what you receive from a single food or a meal, that is most important.

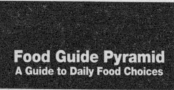

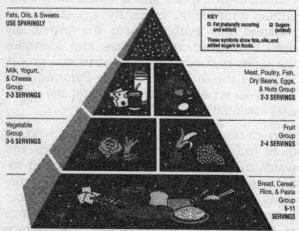

SOURCE: U.S. Department of Agriculture/U.S. Department of Health and Human Services

*The Nutrition Labeling and Education
Act of 1990*

The Nutrition Labeling and Education Act
(NLEA) of l990 requires that the FDA update
labeling regulations for processed food packages. Foods such as meat and poultry are regulated by the U.S. Department of Agriculture,
which voluntarily developed regulations similar to the FDA's for these foods. The NLEA
requires almost all foods to carry nutrition information. Key nutrients like saturated fat
and cholesterol must be included. It ensures
that claims (e.g., "high in fiber" or "helps prevent heart disease") are honest. The new law
also requires the FDA to set standard serving
sizes for l50 food categories. Label information on food packaging is based on serving
size. All serving sizes must be listed in cups,
ounces, teaspoonfuls, tablespoonfuls, or other
standard household measures. Serving sizes
must be the same for similar products and
reflect actual eating habits. Uniform serving
sizes make it easier for consumers to compare
nutritional information.

What does the new nutrition label mean?

The new food package labels tell you how
much of a day's worth (the Daily Value [DV])
of fat, saturated fat, cholesterol, sodium, protein, carbohydrates, vitamin A, vitamin C, calcium, and iron a serving of the food contains.
DVs help you understand how much of a nutrient should be eaten at a minimum (e.g.,
fiber, calcium) or at a maximum (e.g., fat, cholesterol). The DVs listed on the food labels are

based on the needs of people who consume approximately 2000 calories a day (most adults, children, and younger women). Some labels list DVs for 2500 calories a day (younger men, teenage boys, and very active younger women).

The Food Label

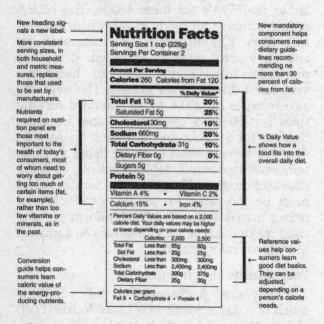

New heading signals a new label. →

More consistent serving sizes, in both household and metric measures, replace those that used to be set by manufacturers.

Nutrients required on nutrition panel are those most important to the health of today's consumers, most of whom need to worry about getting too much of certain items (fat, for example), rather than too few vitamins or minerals, as in the past.

Conversion guide helps consumers learn caloric value of the energy-producing nutrients. →

New mandatory component helps consumers meet dietary guidelines recommending no more than 30 percent of calories from fat.

% Daily Value ← shows how a food fits into the overall daily diet.

Reference values help consumers learn good diet basics. They can be adjusted, depending on a person's calorie needs.

Nutrition Facts
Serving Size 1 cup (228g)
Servings Per Container 2

Amount Per Serving

Calories 260   Calories from Fat 120

	% Daily Value*
Total Fat 13g	**20%**
Saturated Fat 5g	**25%**
Cholesterol 30mg	**10%**
Sodium 660mg	**28%**
Total Carbohydrate 31g	**10%**
Dietary Fiber 0g	**0%**
Sugars 5g	
Protein 5g	

Vitamin A 4%	Vitamin C 2%
Calcium 15%	Iron 4%

* Percent Daily Values are based on a 2,000 calorie diet. Your daily values may be higher or lower depending on your calorie needs:

	Calories:	2,000	2,500
Total Fat	Less than	65g	80g
Sat Fat	Less than	20g	25g
Cholesterol	Less than	300mg	300mg
Sodium	Less than	2,400mg	2,400mg
Total Carbohydrate		300g	375g
Dietary Fiber		25g	30g

Calories per gram:
Fat 9 • Carbohydrate 4 • Protein 4

Food labeling terms defined
Before the passage of the NLEA, food companies did not have to meet any specific require-

ments to label their product as "low fat," "fat free," etc. Therefore, there was little to no uniformity among labeling terms. Since the NLEA, food products must meet specific definitions as outlined by the FDA and the Department of Agriculture before they can make the following claims:

If the label says . . .	Each serving must contain no more than . . .
• Calorie free	• 5 calories
• Low calorie	• 40 calories
• Light or lite	• 1/3 fewer calories or 50% less fat than the standard product
• Fat free	• 1/2 gram of fat
• Low fat	• 3 grams of fat
• Cholesterol free	• 2 milligrams (mg) cholesterol and 2 grams saturated fat
• Low cholesterol	• 20 mg cholesterol and 2 grams saturated fat
• Sodium free	• 5 mg sodium
• Low sodium	• 140 mg sodium
• Healthy	• 480 mg sodium or 95 mg cholesterol (Note that food must also meet the criteria for low fat and saturated fat; it must also have at least 10% DV per serving of vitamin A, vitamin C, calcium, iron, protein, and fiber.)

| • Lean | • 10 grams total fat, 4.5 grams saturated fat, and 95 mg cholesterol (Note that meals and main dishes must meet these criteria per 100 grams of food and per labeled serving; seafood and game meat must meet these criteria per 100 grams of food.) |

Source: Food and Drug Administration, 1993, 1994; U.S. Department of Agriculture, 1994.

Note: These claims have stricter definitions for foods that have small serving sizes. The claims have more lenient definitions for meals and main dishes.

Health claims

Also as part of the NLEA, the FDA now decides what health claims food companies can make to promote their products. The following claims are allowed for foods that meet certain criteria:

- A high calcium intake may reduce the risk of osteoporosis.
- A diet low in sodium reduces the risk of high blood pressure (hypertension).
- A diet low in total fat may reduce the risk of some cancers.
- A diet low in saturated fat and cholesterol may reduce the risk of heart disease.

- A diet high in fruits, vegetables, and some grains may reduce the risk of some cancers.
- A diet high in fruits, vegetables, and some grains may reduce the risk of heart disease.
- A high folic acid intake consumed before conception and during early pregnancy may decrease the risk of having a baby born with serious brain and/or spinal cord defects (neural tube defects).

Source: Food and Drug Administration, 1993.

Daily Recommended Intakes

The daily recommended intakes for vitamins and minerals are defined differently in different countries. For example, in the United States, the Recommended Dietary Allowances (RDAs) for vitamins and minerals are determined by the Food and Nutrition Board (FNB) of the National Research Council (see Tables 1 to 3). They are intended to provide adequate amounts of vitamins and minerals for most healthy persons during normal daily activities. The RDA for a given nutrient may vary depending on a person's age, gender, and physical condition (e.g., pregnancy, breast-feeding). The FDA determines the Daily Value (DV) for a given nutrient based on the range of values provided by the FNB. This is a single value that is used for food labeling. In Canada, these standards are called

Recommended Nutrient Intakes (RNIs) for vitamins and minerals. They are determined by Health and Welfare Canada (see Tables 4 to 6). RNIs provide recommended amounts of each specific nutrient to allow adequate nutrition and lessen the risk of chronic disease.

What Are Vitamins and Minerals and How Do They Work?

Vitamins are compounds that you need in small amounts to remain healthy and function normally. Vitamins do not provide calories; they help the body use proteins, carbohydrates, fats, and minerals. Vitamins are important for such diverse functions as the formation of red blood cells, mental alertness, and helping your body fight infections.

Minerals are elements that are also needed for normal life processes. They are necessary for life and health since they aid a wide variety of body functions, including blood clotting, muscle movements, and fluid balance. In bones, the mineral calcium plays an important structural role. Other minerals such as sodium, sulfur, phosphorus, potassium, magnesium, chloride, iron, manganese, iodine, chromium, fluoride, zinc, cobalt, copper, and selenium are needed in varying amounts.

TABLE 1

FOOD AND NUTRITION BOARD, NATIONAL ACADEMY OF SCIENCES—
NATIONAL RESEARCH COUNCIL RECOMMENDED DIETARY
ALLOWANCES,[a] Revised 1989*
*Designed for the maintenance of good nutrition of practically all healthy
people in the United States*

Age (years) or Condition	Weight[b] (kg)	(lb)	Height[b] (cm)	(in)	C (mg)	Thia-min (mg)	Ribo-flavin (mg)	Niacin (mg NE)[c]	B_6 (mg)	Fo-late (mcg)	B_{12} (mcg)
Infants											
0.0-0.5	6	13	60	24	30	0.3	0.4	5	0.3	25	0.3
0.5-1.0	9	20	71	28	35	0.4	0.5	6	0.6	35	0.5
Children											
1-3	13	29	90	35	40	0.7	0.8	9	1	50	0.7
4-6	20	44	112	44	45	0.9	1.1	12	1.1	75	1
7-10	28	62	132	52	45	1	1.2	13	1.4	100	1.4
Males											
11-14	45	99	157	62	50	1.3	1.5	17	1.7	150	2
15-18	66	145	176	69	60	1.5	1.8	20	2	200	2
19-24	72	160	177	70	60	1.5	1.7	19	2	200	2
25-50	79	174	176	70	60	1.5	1.7	19	2	200	2
51+	77	170	173	68	60	1.2	1.4	15	2	200	2
Females											
11-14	46	101	157	62	50	1.1	1.3	15	1.4	150	2
15-18	55	120	163	64	60	1.1	1.3	15	1.5	180	2
19-24	58	128	164	65	60	1.1	1.3	15	1.6	180	2
25-50	63	138	163	64	60	1.1	1.3	15	1.6	180	2
51+	65	143	160	63	60	1	1.2	13	1.6	180	2
Pregnant					70	1.5	1.6	17	2.2	400	2.2
Lactating											
1st 6 months					95	1.6	1.8	20	2.1	280	2.6
2nd 6 months					90	1.6	1.7	20	2.1	260	2.6

[a] The allowances, expressed as average daily intakes over time, are intended to provide for individual variations among most normal persons as they live in the United States under usual environmental stresses. Diets should be based on a variety of common foods in order to provide other nutrients for which human requirements have been less well defined.

[b] Weights and heights of Reference Adults are actual medians for the U.S. population of the designated age, as reported by National Health and Nutrition Examination Survey II (NHANES II). The median weights and heights of those under 19 years of age were taken from Hamill et al. (1979). The use of these figures does not imply that the height-to-weight ratios are ideal.

[c] 1 NE (niacin equivalent) is equal to 1 milligram (mg) of niacin or 60 mg of dietary tryptophan.

* Reprinted with permission from RECOMMENDED DIETARY ALLOWANCES: 10TH EDITION. Copyright 1989 by the National Academy of Sciences. Courtesy of the National Academy Press, Washington, D.C.

TABLE 2

FOOD AND NUTRITION BOARD, NATIONAL ACADEMY OF SCIENCES—
NATIONAL RESEARCH COUNCIL RECOMMENDED DIETARY
ALLOWANCES,[a] Revised 1989*

*Designed for the maintenance of good nutrition of practically all healthy
people in the United States*

Age (years) or Condition	Weight[b] (kg)	Weight[b] (lb)	Height[b] (cm)	Height[b] (in)	Fat-soluble Vitamins A (mcg RE)[c]	D (mcg)[d]	E (mg alpha-TE)[e]	K (mcg)
Infants								
0.0-0.5	6	13	60	24	375	7.5	3	5
0.5-1.0	9	20	71	28	375	10	4	10
Children								
1-3	13	29	90	35	400	10	6	15
4-6	20	44	112	44	500	10	7	20
7-10	28	62	132	52	700	10	7	30
Males								
11-14	45	99	157	62	1000	10	10	45
15-18	66	145	176	69	1000	10	10	65
19-24	72	160	177	70	1000	10	10	70
25-50	79	174	176	70	1000	5	10	80
51 +	77	170	173	68	1000	5	10	80
Females								
11-14	46	101	157	62	800	10	8	45
15-18	55	120	163	64	800	10	8	55
19-24	58	128	164	65	800	10	8	60
25-50	63	138	163	64	800	5	8	65
51 +	65	143	160	63	800	5	8	65
Pregnant					800	10	10	65
Lactating								
1st 6 months					1300	10	12	65
2nd 6 months					1200	10	11	65

[a] The allowances, expressed as average daily intakes over time, are intended to provide for individual variations among most normal persons as they live in the United States under usual environmental stresses. Diets should be based on a variety of common foods in order to provide other nutrients for which human requirements have been less well defined.

[b] Weights and heights of Reference Adults are actual medians for the U.S. population of the designated age, as reported by National Health and Nutrition Examination Survey II (NHANES II). The median weights and heights of those under 19 years of age were taken from Hamill et al. (1979). The use of these figures does not imply that the height-to-weight ratios are ideal.

[c] Retinol equivalents. 1 retinol equivalent = 1 mcg retinol or 6 mcg beta-carotene.

[d] As cholecalciferol. 10 mcg cholecalciferol = 400 IU of vitamin D.

[e] alpha-Tocopherol equivalents. 1 mg d-alpha tocopherol = 1 alpha-TE.

* Reprinted with permission from RECOMMENDED DIETARY ALLOWANCES: 10TH EDITION. Copyright 1989 by the National Academy of Sciences. Courtesy of the National Academy Press, Washington, D.C.

TABLE 3

FOOD AND NUTRITION BOARD, NATIONAL ACADEMY OF SCIENCES—
NATIONAL RESEARCH COUNCIL RECOMMENDED DIETARY
ALLOWANCES,' Revised 1989*
*Designed for the maintenance of good nutrition of practically all healthy
people in the United States*

Age (years) or Condition	Weight[b] (kg)	(lb)	Height (cm)	(in)	Minerals Calcium (mg)	Phosphorus (mg)	Magnesium (mg)	Iron (mg)	Zinc (mg)	Iodine (mcg)	Selenium (mcg)
Infants											
0.0-0.5	6	13	60	24	400	300	40	6	5	40	10
0.5-1.0	9	20	71	28	600	500	60	10	5	50	15
Children											
1-3	13	29	90	35	800	800	80	10	10	70	20
4-6	20	44	112	44	800	800	120	10	10	90	20
7-10	28	62	132	52	800	800	170	10	10	120	30
Males											
11-14	45	99	157	62	1200	1200	270	12	15	150	40
15-18	66	145	176	69	1200	1200	400	12	15	150	50
19-24	72	160	177	70	1200	1200	350	10	15	150	70
25-50	79	174	176	70	800	800	350	10	15	150	70
51 +	77	170	173	68	800	800	350	10	15	150	70
Females											
11-14	46	101	157	62	1200	1200	280	15	12	150	45
15-18	55	120	163	64	1200	1200	300	15	12	150	50
19-24	58	128	164	65	1200	1200	280	15	12	150	55
25-50	63	138	163	64	800	800	280	15	12	150	55
51 +	65	143	160	63	800	800	280	10	12	150	55
Pregnant					1200	1200	320	30	15	175	65
Lactating											
1st 6 months					1200	1200	355	15	19	200	75
2nd 6 months					1200	1200	340	15	16	200	75

[a] The allowances, expressed as average daily intakes over time, are intended to provide for individual variations among most normal persons as they live in the United States under usual environmental stresses. Diets should be based on a variety of common foods in order to provide other nutrients for which human requirements have been less well defined.

[b] Weights and heights of Reference Adults are actual medians for the U.S. population of the designated age, as reported by National Health and Nutrition Examination Survey II (NHANES II). The median weights and heights of those under 19 years of age were taken from Hamill et al. (1979). The use of these figures does not imply that the height-to-weight ratios are ideal.

* Reprinted with permission from RECOMMENDED DIETARY ALLOWANCES: 10TH EDITION. Copyright 1989 by the National Academy of Sciences. Courtesy of the National Academy Press, Washington, D.C.

TABLE 4

NUTRITION RECOMMENDATIONS—HEALTH AND WELFARE
CANADA, Revised 1990*

Age or Condition	Weight (kg)	Water-soluble Vitamins					
		C (mg)	Thia-min[a] (mg)	Ribo-flavin[a] (mg)	Niacin[a] (NE)[d]	Fo-late (mcg)	B$_{12}$ (mcg)
Infants (months)							
0-4	6	20	0.3	0.3	4	50	0.3
5-12	9	20	0.4	0.5	7	50	0.3
Children (years)							
1	11	20	0.5	0.6	8	65	0.3
2-3	14	20	0.6	0.7	9	80	0.4
4-6	18	25	0.7	0.9	13	90	0.5
Males (years)							
7-9	25	25	0.9	1.1	16	125	0.8
10-12	34	25	1	1.3	18	170	1
13-15	50	30	1.1	1.4	20	150	1.5
16-18	62	40[b]	1.3	1.6	23	185	1.9
19-24	71	40[b]	1.2	1.5	22	210	2
25-49	74	40[b]	1.1	1.4	19	220	2
50-74	73	40[b]	0.9	1.3	16	220	2
75+	69	40[b]	0.8	1	14	205	2
Females (years)							
7-9	25	25	0.8	1	14	125	0.8
10-12	36	25	0.9	1.1	16	180	1
13-15	48	30	0.9	1.1	16	145	1.5
16-18	53	30[b]	0.8	1.1	15	160	1.9
19-24	58	30[b]	0.8	1.1	15	175	2
25-49	59	30[b]	0.8	1	14	175	2
50-74	63	30[b]	0.8[c]	1[c]	14[c]	190	2
75+	64	30[b]	0.8[c]	1[c]	14[c]	190	2
Pregnancy (additional)							
1st Trimester		0	0.1	0.1	0.1	300	1
2nd Trimester		10	0.1	0.3	0.2	300	1
3rd Trimester		10	0.1	0.3	0.2	300	1
Lactation (additional)		25	0.2	0.4	0.3	100	0.5

[a] Nutrient intake based on amount of kcal consumed.
[b] Smokers should increase Vitamin C by 50%.
[c] Level below which intake should not fall.
[d] Niacin equivalents.
* Health Canada, *Nutrition Recommendations: The Report of the Scientific Review Committee 1990*. Reproduced with the permission of the Minister of Supply and Services Canada, 1995.

TABLE 5

NUTRITION RECOMMENDATIONS—HEALTH AND
WELFARE CANADA, Revised 1990*

Age or Condition	Weight (kg)	Fat-soluble Vitamins		
		A (RE)'	D (mcg)	E (mg)
Infants (months)				
0-4	6	400	10	3
5-12	9	400	10	3
Children (years)				
1	11	400	10	3
2-3	14	400	5	4
4-6	18	500	5	5
Males (years)				
7-9	25	700	2.5	7
10-12	34	800	2.5	8
13-15	50	900	5	9
16-18	62	1000	5	10
19-24	71	1000	2.5	10
25-49	74	1000	2.5	9
50-74	73	1000	5	7
75+	69	1000	5	6
Females (years)				
7-9	25	700	2.5	6
10-12	36	800	5	7
13-15	48	800	5	7
16-18	53	800	2.5	7
19-24	58	800	2.5	7
25-49	59	800	2.5	6
50-74	63	800	5	6
75+	64	800	5	5
Pregnancy (additional)				
1st Trimester		100	2.5	2
2nd Trimester		100	2.5	2
3rd Trimester		100	2.5	2
Lactation (additional)		400	2.5	3

ᵃ Retinol equivalents.

* Health Canada, *Nutrition Recommendations: The Report of the Scientific Review Committee 1990.* Reproduced with the permission of the Minister of Supply and Services Canada, 1995.

TABLE 6

NUTRITION RECOMMENDATIONS—HEALTH AND WELFARE CANADA,
Revised 1990*

Age or Condition	Weight (kg)	Calcium (mg)	Phos-phorus (mg)	Mag-nesium (mg)	Iron (mg)	Iodine (mcg)	Zinc (mg)
Infants (months)							
0-4	6	250[a]	150	20	0.3[b]	30	2[b]
5-12	9	400	200	32	7	40	3
Children (years)							
1	11	500	300	40	6	55	4
2-3	14	550	350	50	6	65	4
4-6	18	600	400	65	8	85	5
Males (years)							
7-9	25	700	500	100	8	110	7
10-12	34	900	700	130	8	125	9
13-15	50	1100	900	185	10	160	12
16-18	62	900	1000	230	10	160	12
19-24	71	800	1000	240	9	160	12
25-49	74	800	1000	250	9	160	12
50-74	73	800	1000	250	9	160	12
75+	69	800	1000	230	9	160	12
Females (years)							
7-9	25	700	500	100	8	95	7
10-12	36	1100	800	135	8	110	9
13-15	48	1000	850	180	13	160	9
16-18	53	700	850	200	12	160	9
19-24	58	700	850	200	13	160	9
25-49	59	700	850	200	13	160	9
50-74	63	800	850	210	8	160	9
75+	64	800	850	210	8	160	9
Pregnancy (additional)							
1st Trimester		500	200	15	0	25	6
2nd Trimester		500	200	45	5	25	6
3rd Trimester		500	200	45	10	25	6
Lactation (additional)		500	200	65	0	50	6

[a] Infant formula with high phosphorus should contain 375 mg calcium.
[b] Breast milk is assumed to be the source of the mineral.
* Health Canada, *Nutrition Recommendations: The Report of the Scientific Review Committee 1990.* Reproduced with the permission of the Minister of Supply and Services Canada, 1995.

ABOUT DIETARY
SUPPLEMENTS

Fat-Soluble Versus
Water-Soluble Vitamins

At this time, thirteen essential vitamins have been identified. Each of these vitamins is soluble either in water or in fat. The fat-soluble vitamins are vitamins A, D, E, and K. In addition, beta-carotene is a fat-soluble nutrient that is changed to vitamin A in the body. Water-soluble vitamins are vitamin C and the B complex vitamins, which include vitamin B_1 (thiamine), B_2 (riboflavin), B_3 (niacin), B_5 (pantothenic acid), B_6 (pyridoxine), B_{12} (cyanocobalamin), biotin, and folic acid.

Fat-soluble vitamins are stored in the body. Therefore, you are more likely to accumulate toxic amounts, especially with high doses of vitamins A and D. Fat-soluble vitamins are not easily destroyed by heat in cooking or processing or through exposure to air.

Water-soluble vitamins are stored in the body in small amounts and are less likely to accumulate in toxic concentrations. They are termed water-soluble vitamins because they dissolve easily in water. However, deficiencies of water-soluble vitamins develop faster than do deficiencies of fat-soluble vitamins. Surpluses of most water-soluble vitamins are eliminated in the urine, but excesses of some can cause harm. For example, women who took large amounts (more than 200 to 500 milligrams a day) of vitamin B_6 developed symptoms of nerve damage that disappeared when they stopped taking it.

Are Natural Vitamins Better Than Synthetic Vitamins?

With the exception of vitamin E, there is no evidence to suggest that natural vitamins are, in any way, better than synthetic vitamins. In fact, it has not been proven that the body reacts differently to a natural than a synthetic vitamin. Natural and synthetic vitamins perform the same functions, and usually with the same efficiency. The only exception is natural vitamin E (d-alpha tocopherol), which may be better used by the body than synthetic vitamin E. Unfortunately, the word "natural" on the label of a vitamin E product does not guarantee that the vitamin E contained in that product is the all-natural form.

Natural vitamins are derived from substances found in nature. For example, natural beta-carotene may come from algae or vegetable sources, natural vitamin E may come from vegetable oil, and natural vitamin C may come from rose hips. Some products that are labeled "natural" are mostly synthetic vitamins that have been mixed with plant extracts or tiny amounts of natural vitamins. The so-called natural products go through most of the same "unnatural" processing procedures that the synthetic ones go through.

Natural calcium products derived from bone meal or dolomite could be dangerous because they may contain too much lead.

Although products claim to include different ingredients, there are a few important things to remember. First, a vitamin is a vitamin, no matter where it comes from. Chemically, there is no difference between a vitamin derived from plants or other substances found in nature and a vitamin made synthetically. All dietary supplement makers buy most of their raw materials and minerals from the same source. Higher cost of a product may not necessarily indicate higher quality.

Who Needs Vitamins and Minerals?

Despite supplementing the food supply with some nutrients, vitamin and/or mineral deficiencies may be caused by improper dietary practices that extend over a long period of time. Certain diseases or medications you may be taking may also cause a deficiency. Still other people may not absorb from their diet the nutrients they need.

In general, there are several basic ways a person may become nutrient deficient. These include:

Inadequate intake (e.g., anorexics, dieters, the elderly, vegetarians)

Improper absorption (e.g., alcoholics, the elderly, patients with gastrointestinal diseases or malabsorption syndromes)

Increased requirements (e.g., pregnant women, breast-feeding women, cigarette smokers, premature infants, renal patients, certain long-term medication users)

Increased losses (e.g., patients with bulimia or diarrhea, certain long-term medication users)

The following are considerations for specific age groups or patient conditions:

Babies—Low-birth-weight babies (babies weighing less than 5.5 pounds at birth) may be deficient in some nutrients. Because they have periods of rapid growth, normal-weight babies may need extra supplementation. Some infant feeding practices (e.g., the use of goat's milk or powdered milk) may not provide all nutrients needed. Your health care professional may recommend that you change your feeding practice to use an infant formula or that your baby receive a dietary supplement. Many health care professionals recommend vitamins A and D and fluoride for breast-fed babies.

Teenagers—Some teenagers may be deficient in certain nutrients because they have periods of rapid growth and may not eat properly. Iron deficiency may be a problem in teenage girls especially.

Women of childbearing age—Due to heavy blood loss from menstruation, many women of premenopausal age may need iron supplementation. In addition, it is important that women planning to become pregnant consume a total of 400 micrograms (0.4 mg) of folic acid a day from food and supplements. This will reduce the risk of having a baby born with serious brain and/or spinal cord defects (neural tube defects). Neural tube defects include spina bifida (an imperfect closure of the spinal column) and anencephalitis (little or no brain tissue). It is important that folic acid be taken regularly before becoming pregnant to prevent possible neural tube defects.

Pregnant women—The need for most vitamins and minerals is increased during pregnancy. Your health care professional may recommend a dietary supplement, especially one containing iron and folic acid. As mentioned above, it is important that you continue to consume enough folic acid throughout pregnancy. Discuss your nutritional needs with your doctor or health care professional if you are pregnant.

Breast-feeding—The need for most vitamins and minerals is increased during breast-feeding. If certain vitamins or minerals are deficient in a nursing mother's diet, they will be deficient in her breast milk as well. Many health care professionals recommend that breast-feeding women take a prenatal multivitamin and mineral supplement. However, taking large amounts of a dietary supplement while breast-feeding may be harmful to the mother and/or baby and should be avoided unless prescribed by your health care professional.

Long-term medicine and dietary supplement users—Use of some medicines or certain dietary supplements for long periods of time may deprive the body of essential nutrients. You may want to discuss your nutritional needs with your health care professional.

Selected medicines, foods, or dietary supplements used long-term that may increase required amounts of specific nutrients (Note: An asterisk [*] indicates those medicines/dietary supplements that may cause more serious nutritional needs):

Medicine/Food/Dietary Supplement	Nutrient (increased need for)
Mineral oil Neomycin	Beta-carotene
*Phytate (as found in wheat bran) Sodium fluoride	Calcium
*Penicillamine (e.g., Cuprimine, Depen) *Zinc supplements	Copper
Analgesics *Antacids Anticonvulsants (seizure medicine) Epoetin (e.g., Epogen, Eprex, Procrit) Estrogens	Folic acid

Medicine/Food/Dietary Supplement	Nutrient (increased need for)
Histamine H_2-receptor antagonists (e.g., Axid, Pepcid, Tagamet, Zantac) Sulfasalazine (e.g., Azulfidine) Zinc supplements	
Antacids *Calcium supplements Epoetin (e.g., Epogen, Eprex, Procrit) *Penicillamine (e.g., Cuprimine, Depen) *Phytate (as found in wheat bran) Trientine (e.g., Syprine) *Zinc supplements	Iron
Cisplatin (e.g., Platinol) Cyclosporine (e.g., Sandimmune) Gentamicin (e.g., Garamycin) *Digitalis medicines (heart medicines) Loop diuretics (water pills) Thiazide diuretics (water pills) Etidronate (e.g., Didronel) Sodium polystyrene sulfonate (e.g., Kayexalate)	Magnesium
Antacids Iron supplements Zinc supplements	Phosphates

Medicine/Food/Dietary Supplement	Nutrient (increased need for)
*Amphotericin B (e.g., Fungizone)	Potassium
Corticosteroids	
Corticotropin	
Polymyxin B	
*Thiazide diuretics (water pills)	
Insulin	
Sodium bicarbonate (baking soda)	
Laxatives	
*Cycloserine (e.g., Seromycin)	Pyridoxine
*Ethionamide (e.g., Trecator-SC)	
Hydralazine (e.g., Apresoline)	
Immunosuppressants	
*Isoniazid (e.g., Laniazid, Nydrazid)	
Penicillamine (e.g., Cuprimine, Depen)	
Oral contraceptives	
Tricyclic antidepressants (medicines for depression)	Riboflavin
Phenothiazines	
Probenecid (e.g., Benemid)	
Aluminum hydroxide (found in some antacids)	Sodium fluoride
Calcium supplements	
Mineral oil	Vitamin A
Neomycin	
Epoetin (e.g., Epogen, Eprex, Procrit)	Vitamin B_{12}
*Omeprazole (e.g., Prilosec)	

Medicine/Food/Dietary Supplement	Nutrient (increased need for)
Barbiturates	Vitamin D
Cholestyramine (e.g., Questran)	
Colestipol (e.g., Colestid)	
Hydantoin anticonvulsants (seizure medicines)	
Mineral oil	
Primidone (e.g., Myidone, Mysoline)	
Mineral oil	Vitamin E
Iron supplements	
Antacids	Vitamin K
Antibiotics (broad spectrum)	
Quinidine (e.g., Quinidex Extentabs)	
Quinine (e.g., Quinamm)	
Salicylates (high doses)	
Mineral oil	
Sucralfate (e.g., Carafate)	
Vitamin E supplements	
*Calcium supplements	Zinc
*Folic acid supplements	
Penicillamine (e.g., Cuprimine, Depen)	
*Iron supplements	
*Phytate (as found in wheat bran)	
Thiazide diuretics (water pills)	
Phosphorus-containing medicines	

Claims Made for Vitamins and Minerals

Many people who take a vitamin and/or mineral supplement do so to protect themselves against deficiencies. Others may take dietary supplements because of what they hear on television or from friends or what they read in newspapers or magazines. Ads for dietary supplements may claim that they are beneficial to prevent or treat balding, to cure AIDS, or to live longer. Lately, claims have been made for the antioxidants (e.g., vitamins C, E, and beta-carotene), and their potential role in the protection against cancer and heart disease. Many claims have not been proven effective; however, research may be ongoing, as with the antioxidants.

Dietary supplement companies are not allowed to make specific claims (e.g., treatment for baldness, cure for AIDS) for their products unless they have been evaluated and approved by the Food and Drug Administration (FDA). However, they are allowed to make general claims (e.g., strengthens the immune system). To date, the FDA has approved two health claims that affect dietary supplements: adequate calcium intake to reduce the risk of osteoporosis and adequate folic acid intake before and during pregnancy for the prevention of serious brain and/or spinal cord defects (neural tube defects) in babies.

How do I determine that a claim is valid?

In deciding whether to believe a claim about a particular nutrient or dietary supplement, consider the following questions:

- Is the claim based on scientific research?
- Has the information been reviewed by science experts? What are the qualifications of those experts?
- Is publicity being used as evidence?
- Are extraordinary health claims being made for the product?

Other questions you should ask include the following:

- Has the product been proven safe?
- If there is a risk, is the risk justified?
- Is the cost for the product justified?

If you are in doubt about a claim made for a dietary supplement, ask your health care professional for advice.

Can I Take Too Much of a Vitamin or Mineral?

The fat-soluble vitamins (A, D, E, and K) are stored in the body; therefore, when you take more than you need, they will build up in the body. Most water-soluble vitamins are not stored as readily if taken in quantities larger than the recommended daily intake; however, if you take more than you need, the excess will pass into your urine. Taking excessive amounts of some minerals may also cause a buildup in the body. A buildup of vitamins and minerals may lead to severe adverse reactions and in some cases, poisoning.

The following are adverse reactions that have been reported when excess amounts of the specified vitamins or minerals are taken:

- **Vitamin A**—If you take 25,000 Units (IUs) or more daily for several months, liver damage, hair loss, bone pain, blurred vision, and headaches can occur.
- **Vitamin B$_6$**—Doses of 200 to 500 milligrams (mg) a day for several months may cause numbness in the feet and hands and difficulty in walking.
- **Vitamin C**—Doses higher than 1000 mg (1 gram) a day for long periods of time can cause diarrhea.
- **Vitamin D**—Doses higher than 5000 Units a day for several weeks can cause bone pain and the buildup of calcium in the blood, urine, and other body tissues. This may cause constipation, headache, nausea, and kidney stones.
- **Zinc**—Doses higher than 20 mg a day added to the zinc already in your diet should not be taken for longer than one month. Higher doses may cause a deficiency of copper and increased risk of heart disease and anemia.

GENERAL INFORMATION ABOUT USE OF DIETARY SUPPLEMENTS

Proper Use of Your Supplement

If you are taking a dietary supplement at your health care professional's recommendation, take your supplement as directed. If you are taking it on your own, follow the normal daily recommended intake.

Should I take my dietary supplement with meals or on an empty stomach?

- Most dietary supplements can be taken with meals or on an empty stomach. Many people find it easier to remember to take them with meals. However, some nutrients are best taken before or after meals because they are better absorbed.

Missed Dose

If you miss taking a vitamin or mineral for one or more days there is no cause for concern, since it takes some time for your body to become seriously low in vitamins or minerals. However, if your health care professional has recommended that you take a vitamin or mineral, try to remember to take it as directed.

Storage of Your Dietary Supplement

To store your dietary supplement:

- Keep out of reach of children.

- Store away from heat and direct light.
- Do not store capsules or tablets in the bathroom, near the kitchen sink, or in any other damp places. Heat or moisture may cause the dietary supplement to break down.
- Do not keep outdated dietary supplements or those no longer needed. Be sure that any discarded dietary supplement is out of the reach of children.

Communicating with Your Health Care Professional

Purchasing a dietary supplement is a personal decision. In most cases, dietary supplements are not prescribed by a health care professional (e.g., doctor, nurse, pharmacist, dietitian, dentist) and do not require a prescription. However, if you think you are not getting enough of a specific nutrient from the foods you eat, you may want to discuss this with a health care professional, not the salesperson in the store, before selecting a dietary supplement.

If you purchase your dietary supplement in a pharmacy, you may want to have your pharmacist help you choose a product that meets your needs and is of good quality.

Considerations When Choosing a Dietary Supplement

Dietary supplements can be purchased in a variety of ways—pharmacies, health food stores, grocery stores, through the mail, and in many other types of stores. If you buy them in some of these places, you may need to select the dietary supplement on your own. Given all of the choices in the marketplace, this could be difficult. For example, you may decide you want to take vitamin C. A look at the bottles of vitamin C on the shelf may show vitamin C from rose hips, vitamin C with acerola, vitamin C with fruit flavor, extended-release vitamin C, vitamin C plus acerola and bioflavonoids, or vitamin C with natural orange flavor. The following guidelines should be used when selecting your own dietary supplement.

- Unless directed by your health care professional, choose a balanced, multiple-ingredient dietary supplement rather than one with one or two specific nutrients.

- Choose a preparation that provides approximately 50 to 100% of the Daily Value (DV) for recognized nutrients.

- Keep in mind that most dietary supplements do not provide 100% of the DV for calcium because the added calcium would make the supplement too big to swallow easily. If you must take extra calcium, you may need to get it from a separate supplement.

- Claims that a product is "natural," "organic," "therapeutic," "extended-release," or "high potency" may be only advertising gimmicks to make you think the product is better.

- Choose a preparation with an expiration date that is clearly marked and far enough in the future to allow you to use all of the product. Certain vitamins or minerals lose potency with time, especially in hot and humid climates.

- The price of the dietary supplement is not necessarily an indication of the quality of the product.

- If you are concerned about dietary supplement quality, you may want to look for products that meet USP standards. In some cases, this will be stated on the label. However, other products may meet USP standards but do not state it on the label. If you are in doubt, check with your pharmacist.

- If you have allergies, make sure that you read the ingredients section of the dietary supplement label. You may be allergic to other substances in the dietary supplement, such as a preservative, yellow dye, or sulfites.

How To Read A Supplement Label*

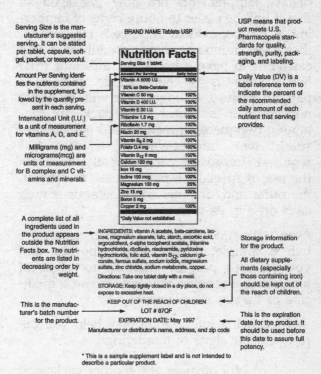

Serving Size is the manufacturer's suggested serving. It can be stated per tablet, capsule, softgel, packet, or teaspoonful.

Amount Per Serving identifies the nutrients contained in the supplement, followed by the quantity present in each serving.

International Unit (I.U.) is a unit of measurement for vitamins A, D, and E.

Milligrams (mg) and micrograms(mcg) are units of measurement for B complex and C vitamins and minerals.

A complete list of all ingredients used in the product appears outside the Nutrition Facts box. The nutrients are listed in decreasing order by weight.

This is the manufacturer's batch number for the product.

USP means that product meets U.S. Pharmacopeia standards for quality, strength, purity, packaging, and labeling.

Daily Value (DV) is a label reference term to indicate the percent of the recommended daily amount of each nutrient that serving provides.

Storage information for the product.

All dietary supplements (especially those containing iron) should be kept out of the reach of children.

This is the expiration date for the product. It should be used before this date to assure full potency.

BRAND NAME Tablets USP

Nutrition Facts

Serving Size 1 tablet:

Amount Per Serving	Daily Value
Vitamin A 5000 I.U.	100%
50% as Beta-Carotene	
Vitamin C 60 mg	100%
Vitamin D 400 I.U.	100%
Vitamin E 30 I.U.	100%
Thiamine 1.5 mg	100%
Riboflavin 1.7 mg	100%
Niacin 20 mg	100%
Vitamin B_6 2 mg	100%
Folate 0.4 mg	100%
Vitamin B_{12} 6 mcg	100%
Calcium 120 mg	10%
Iron 15 mg	100%
Iodine 150 mcg	100%
Magnesium 100 mg	25%
Zinc 15 mg	100%
Boron 5 mg	*
Copper 2 mg	100%

*Daily Value not established

INGREDIENTS: vitamin A acetate, beta-carotene, lactose, magnesium stearate, talc, starch, ascorbic acid, ergocalciferol, d-alpha tocopherol acetate, thiamine hydrochloride, riboflavin, niacinamide, pyridoxine hydrochloride, folic acid, vitamin B_{12}, calcium gluconate, ferrous sulfate, sodium iodide, magnesium sulfate, zinc chloride, sodium metaborate, copper.

Directions: Take one tablet daily with a meal.

STORAGE: Keep tightly closed in a dry place, do not expose to excessive heat.

KEEP OUT OF THE REACH OF CHILDREN

LOT # 87QF

EXPIRATION DATE: May 1997

Manufacturer or distributor's name, address, and zip code

* This is a sample supplement label and is not intended to describe a particular product.

Tips Against Tampering

Over-the-counter (OTC) medicines and some dietary supplements are now packaged so that it will be easier to notice signs of tampering. A tamper-evident package is required either to be unique so that it cannot be copied easily, or to have a barrier or indicator (that has an identifying characteristic, such as a pattern, picture, or logo) that will be easily noticed if it is broken. For packages containing two-piece, unsealed, hard gelatin capsules, two tamper-evident features are required. Improved packaging also includes the use of special wrappers, seals, or caps on the outer and/or inner containers, or sealing each dose in its own pouch.

Even with such packaging, however, no system is completely safe. It is important that you do your part by checking for signs of tampering whenever you buy or use a medicine or dietary supplement.

The following information may help you detect possible signs of tampering:

- *Look very carefully* at the outer packaging of the medicine or dietary supplement product before you buy it. After you buy it, also check the inner packaging as soon as possible.
- *Do not take* medicines or dietary supplements that show even the slightest signs of tampering or don't seem quite right.

- Never take medicines or dietary supplements in the dark or in poor lighting. *Read*, using your eyeglasses if necessary, the label and check each dose of the dietary supplement before you take it.

Whenever you suspect that something is unusual about a medicine or dietary supplement or its packaging, take it to your pharmacist or a salesperson in the store where you purchased it. He or she is familiar with most products and their packaging.

Unintentional Poisoning

According to information provided by the American Association of Poison Control Centers, nearly one million children 6 years of age and under were unintentionally poisoned in 1993. Specifically, accidental poisoning with iron supplements has been on the rise. Since 1986, reports have been received of 110,000 children accidentally swallowing iron tablets, resulting in 33 deaths. Taking excess amounts of other dietary supplements, such as selenium, can result in poisoning as well.

If you think you or your child has received an overdose of a medicine or dietary supplement, contact your physician or local Poison Control Center at once.

Dietary Supplement Monographs

Entries appear alphabetically by generic or "family" names. To find the location of brand name entries, refer to the Index at the back of the book.

ASCORBIC ACID (Vitamin C)
Systemic

Some commonly used brand names are:

In the U.S.—

Ascorbicap	Cetane
Cebid Timecelles	Cevi-Bid
Cecon	Flavorcee
Cecore 500	Mega-C/A Plus
Cee-500	Ortho/CS
Cemill	Sunkist
Cenolate	

Generic name product may also be available.

In Canada—

Apo-C	Ce-Vi-Sol

Generic name product may also be available.

Another commonly used name is Vitamin C.

Description

Vitamins (VYE-ta-mins) are compounds that you *must* have for growth and health. They are needed in small amounts only and are usually available in the foods that you eat. Ascorbic (a-SKOR-bik) acid, also known as vitamin C, is necessary for wound healing. It is needed for many functions in the body, including the use of carbohydrates and to help make fats and protein. Vitamin C strengthens blood vessel walls.

Lack of vitamin C can lead to a condition called scurvy, which causes muscle weakness, swollen and bleeding gums, loss of teeth, and bleeding under the skin, as well as tiredness and depression. Wounds also do not heal easily. Your health care professional may treat scurvy by prescribing vitamin C for you.

Increased need for vitamin C may occur in patients with the following conditions:

• AIDS (acquired immune deficiency syndrome)
• Alcoholism
• Burns
• Cancer
• Diarrhea (prolonged)
• Fever (prolonged)
• Infection (prolonged)
• Intestinal diseases
• Overactive thyroid (hyperthyroidism)
• Stomach ulcer
• Stress (continuing)
• Surgical removal of stomach
• Tuberculosis

Also, the following groups of people may have a deficiency of vitamin C:

• Infants receiving unfortified formulas
• Smokers
• Patients using an artificial kidney (on hemodialysis)
• Patients who undergo surgery
• Individuals who are exposed to long periods of cold temperatures

Increased need for vitamin C should be determined by your health care professional.

Injectable vitamin C is administered only by

or under the supervision of your health care professional. Other forms of vitamin C are available without a prescription.

Vitamin C is available in the following dosage forms:

Oral

- Extended-release capsules (U.S.)
- Oral solution (U.S. and Canada)
- Syrup (U.S.)
- Tablets (U.S. and Canada)
- Chewable tablets (U.S. and Canada)
- Effervescent tablets (U.S.)
- Extended-release tablets (U.S. and Canada)

Parenteral

- Injection (U.S.)

Importance of Diet

Vitamin C is found in various foods, including citrus fruits (oranges, lemons, grapefruit), green vegetables (peppers, broccoli, cabbage), tomatoes, and potatoes. It is best to eat fresh fruits and vegetables whenever possible since they contain the most vitamins. Food processing may destroy some of the vitamins. For example, exposure to air, drying, salting, or cooking (especially in copper pots), mincing of fresh vegetables, or mashing potatoes may reduce the amount of vitamin C in foods. Freezing does not usually cause loss of vitamin C unless foods are stored for a very long time.

Normal daily recommended intakes in milligrams (mg) for vitamin C are generally defined as follows:

Persons	U.S. (mg)	Canada (mg)
Infants and children		
Birth to 3 years of age	30–40	20
4 to 6 years of age	45	25
7 to 10 years of age	45	25
Adolescent and adult males	50–60	25–40
Adolescent and adult females	50–60	25–30
Pregnant females	70	30–40
Breast-feeding females	90–95	55
Smokers	100	45–60

Before Using This Dietary Supplement

If you are taking this dietary supplement without a prescription, carefully read and follow any precautions on the label. For vitamin C, the following should be considered:

Pregnancy—Taking too much vitamin C daily throughout pregnancy may possibly harm the fetus.

Breast-feeding—You should check with your health care professional if you are giving your baby an unfortified formula. In that case, the baby must get the vitamins needed some other way.

Other medical problems—The presence of other medical problems may affect the use of vitamin C. Make sure you tell your health care professional if you have any other medical problems, especially:

- Blood problems—High doses of vitamin C may cause certain blood problems
- Diabetes mellitus (sugar diabetes)—Very high doses of vitamin C may interfere with tests for sugar in the urine
- Glucose-6-phosphate dehydrogenase (G6PD) deficiency—High doses of vitamin C may cause hemolytic anemia
- Kidney stones (history of)—High doses of vitamin C may increase risk of kidney stones in the urinary tract

---

Proper Use of This Dietary Supplement

For those individuals taking the *oral liquid form* of vitamin C:

- This preparation is to be taken by mouth even though it comes in a dropper bottle.
- This dietary supplement may be dropped directly into the mouth or mixed with cereal, fruit juice, or other food.

Precautions While Using This Dietary Supplement

Vitamin C is not stored in the body. If you take more than you need, the extra vitamin C will pass into your urine. Very large doses may also interfere with tests for sugar in diabetics and with tests for blood in the stool.

Side Effects of This Dietary Supplement

Along with its needed effects, a dietary supplement may cause some unwanted effects. Although not all of these side effects may occur, if they do occur, they may need medical attention.

Check with your health care professional as soon as possible if the following side effect occurs:

Less common or rare—with high doses
Side or lower back pain

Other side effects may occur that usually do not need medical attention. These side effects may go away during treatment as your body adjusts to the dietary supplement. However, check with your health care professional as soon as possible if any of the following side effects continue or are bothersome:

Less common or rare—with high doses
Diarrhea; dizziness or faintness (with the injection only); flushing or redness of skin; headache; increase in urination (mild); nausea or vomiting; stomach cramps

Other side effects not listed above may also occur in some individuals. If you notice any other effects, check with your health care professional.

Other Claimed Uses

Claims that vitamin C is effective for preventing senility and for treating asthma, some mental problems, cancer, hardening of the arteries, allergies, eye ulcers, blood clots, gum disease, and pressure sores have not been proven. Although vitamin C is being used to reduce the risk of cardiovascular disease, there is not enough information to show that this is effective.

Vitamin C and Cancer

Claimed use: Some people think that taking vitamin C supplements may be useful in reducing the risk of cancer.

Possible action: Vitamin C may reduce the risk of cancer by protecting the body from unstable molecules known as free radicals. Free radicals are molecules that result from natural body processes. It is believed that by a process called oxidation, free radicals damage the body's cells. This is thought to be one of the many possible causes of cancer. As an antioxidant, vitamin C binds to free radicals and makes them inactive.

Current findings: The results of one study involving 30,000 adults in Linxian, China, became available in 1993. After five years, those who took a daily supplement of vitamin C (120 milligrams [mg]) had the same cancer rate as those who took a pill that did not contain vitamin C (placebo).

Role of diet: It has been well documented that people who consume diets high in fruits and vegetables have a decreased risk of certain cancers, especially colon, stomach, esophagus, and oral cancers. Fruits and vegetables are rich in vitamin C as well as other antioxidants.

Conclusion: Based on the results of the Linxian, China, study, taking vitamin C supplements to reduce the risk of cancer cannot be recommended. Results from several large studies should give us more information over the next few years. In the meantime, increasing the amount of fruits and vegetables in your diet appears to be one of many life-style changes that may reduce your risk of developing cancer.

Additional reading: The Linxian, China, study can be found in the *Journal of the National Cancer Institute*, 1993, Volume 85, pages 1483-1492. Additional information on vitamin C can be found in the following publications: *Consumer Reports on Health,* March 1994, pages 25-27; *Nutrition Action Healthletter*, November 1994, pages 10-11.

Vitamin C and the Common Cold

Claimed use: Some people think that taking vitamin C may be useful in preventing or treating the common cold.

Possible action: Vitamin C may play a role in your body's immune response. Your immune response is triggered when you are exposed to substances that cause a cold.

Current findings: Many studies have found that vitamin C does not prevent the common cold. However, a few studies have shown that vitamin C may slightly reduce the length of a cold and make the symptoms (cough, fever, chills, runny nose) less severe. Most studies used doses of 1 to 3 grams of vitamin C per day, taken for two to nine months.

Conclusion: There is no scientific evidence to support use of vitamin C for the prevention of the common cold. However, many people continue to take vitamin C during the cold season. If you take more vitamin C than you need, it will simply be eliminated from your body. Taking doses of vitamin C greater than 1 gram per day for long periods of time has been reported to cause diarrhea. Very high doses of vitamin C may interfere with tests for sugar in the urine.

Additional reading: More information on vitamin C can be found in *Consumer Reports on Health,* January 1995, pages 8-9; and in the *Nutrition Action Healthletter,* November 1994, pages 10-11.

BETA-CAROTENE—For Dietary Supplement (Vitamin) Systemic

Some commonly used brand names are:

In the U.S.—

Max-Caro   Solatene

Provatene

Generic name product is also available.

In Canada—

Generic name product is available.

Description

Beta-carotene (bay-ta-KARE-oh-teen) is converted in the body to vitamin A, which is necessary for normal growth and health and for healthy eyes and skin.

In the absence of a dietary source of vitamin A, a lack of beta-carotene may also lead to a deficiency of vitamin A, which may cause a rare condition called night blindness (problems seeing in the dark). It may also cause dry eyes, eye infections, skin problems, and slowed growth. Your health care professional may treat these problems by prescribing beta-carotene or vitamin A for you.

Some conditions may increase your need for beta-carotene or vitamin A. These include:

- Cystic fibrosis
- Diarrhea, continuing
- Illness, long-term

13

- Injury, serious
- Liver disease
- Malabsorption problems
- Pancreas disease

Increased needed for beta-carotene or vitamin A should be determined by your health care professional.

Beta-carotene is available without a prescription in the following dosage forms:

Oral

- Capsules (U.S. and Canada)
- Tablets (U.S. and Canada)
- Chewable tablets (Canada)

Importance of Diet

Beta-carotene is found in carrots; dark-green leafy vegetables, such as spinach, green leafy lettuce; tomatoes; sweet potatoes; broccoli; cantaloupe; and winter squash. The body converts beta-carotene into vitamin A. Ordinary cooking does not destroy beta-carotene.

Normal daily recommended intakes for beta-carotene are generally defined as follows:

- Children—3 to 6 milligrams (mg) of beta-carotene (the equivalent of 5000 to 10,000 Units of vitamin A activity).

- Adults and adolescents—6 to 15 mg of beta-carotene (the equivalent of 10,000 to 25,000 Units of vitamin A activity).

Before Using This Dietary Supplement

If you are taking this dietary supplement without a prescription, carefully read and follow any precautions on the label. For beta-carotene, the following should be considered:

Pregnancy—Beta-carotene has not been studied in pregnant women. However, no problems with fertility or pregnancy have been reported in women taking up to 30 milligrams (mg) (50,000 Units of vitamin A activity) of beta-carotene a day. The effects of taking more than 30 mg (50,000 Units of vitamin A activity) a day are not known.

Other medical problems—The presence of other medical problems may affect the use of beta-carotene. Make sure you tell your health care professional if you have any other medical problems, especially:

- Kidney disease or
- Liver disease—These conditions may cause high blood levels of beta-carotene, which may increase the chance of side effects

Proper Use of This Dietary Supplement

Beta-carotene is safer than vitamin A (retinol) because vitamin A can be harmful in high doses. If you have high blood levels of vitamin A, then your body will convert less beta-carotene to vitamin A. However, you should take large doses of beta-carotene only under the direction of your health care professional after need has been identified.

Side Effects of This Dietary Supplement

Along with its needed effects, a dietary supplement may cause some unwanted effects. The following side effects may go away during treatment as your body adjusts to the dietary supplement. However, check with your health care professional if any of the following side effects continue or are bothersome:

More common

> Yellowing of palms, hand, or soles of feet, and to a lesser extent the face (this may be a sign that your dose of beta-carotene as a dietary supplement is too high)

Rare

> Diarrhea; dizziness; joint pain; unusual bleeding or bruising

Other side effects not listed above may also occur in some individuals. If you notice any other effects, check with your health care professional.

Other Claimed Uses

Claims that beta-carotene or vitamin A is effective as a sunscreen have not been proven.

Beta-Carotene and Cancer

Claimed use: Some people think that taking

beta-carotene supplements may be useful in reducing the risk of cancer.

Possible action: Some beta-carotene is converted to vitamin A in the body. It is thought that beta-carotene not converted to vitamin A may reduce the risk of cancer by protecting the body from unstable molecules known as free radicals. Free radicals are molecules that result from natural body processes. It is believed that by a process called oxidation, free radicals damage the body's cells. This is thought to be one of the many possible causes of cancer. As an antioxidant, beta-carotene binds to free radicals and renders them inactive.

Current findings: The results from two major studies have become available over the past few years. One study involved 30,000 adults in Linxian, China. After five years, the group receiving daily supplements of beta-carotene (15 milligrams [mg]), vitamin E (30 mg), and selenium (50 micrograms [mcg]) had a lower rate of cancer, especially stomach cancer. However, another study of 29,000 male smokers in Finland actually found an 18% increase in lung cancer in the group receiving 20 mg of beta-carotene a day for five to eight years.

Role of diet: It has been well documented that people who consume diets high in fruits and vegetables have a decreased risk of various cancers, especially lung, colon, stomach, esophagus, and oral cancers. Fruits and vegetables are rich in beta-carotene as well as other antioxidants.

Conclusion: The Linxian study took place in an area of China where a high rate of malnutrition and stomach cancer exists. Therefore, many researchers are not ready to assume that beta-carotene prevents cancer in the U.S. In addition, three supplements with antioxidant properties (beta-carotene, selenium, and vitamin E) were taken together, making it difficult to separate any one as having a positive influence by itself. Results from several large studies using beta-carotene supplements should be available over the next few years. In the meantime, increasing the amount of fruits and vegetables in your diet appears to be one of many life-style changes that may reduce your risk of developing cancer.

Additional reading: The Linxian, China, study can be found in the *Journal of the National Cancer Institute,* 1993, Volume 85, pages 1483-1492. The Finnish study can be found in the *New England Journal of Medicine,* 1994, Volume 330, pages 1029-1035. Additional information on beta-carotene can be found in the following publications: *Consumer Reports on Health,* August 1994, pages 85-88; *Nutrition Action Healthletter,* January/February 1995, pages 8-9.

BIOTIN   Systemic

Generic name product is available in the U.S. and Canada.

Other commonly used names are vitamin H, coenzyme R, or vitamin Bw.

Description

Biotin (BYE-oh-tin) supplements are used to prevent or treat biotin deficiency.

Vitamins (VYE-ta-mins) are compounds that you must have for growth and health. They are needed in only small amounts and are usually available in the foods that you eat. Biotin is necessary for formation of fatty acids and glucose, which are used as fuels by the body. It is also important for the metabolism of amino acids and carbohydrates.

A lack of biotin is rare. However, if it occurs, it may lead to skin rash, loss of hair, high blood levels of cholesterol, and heart problems.

Some conditions may increase your need for biotin. These include:

- Genetic disorder of biotin deficiency
- Seborrheic dermatitis in infants
- Surgical removal of the stomach

Increased need for biotin should be determined by your health care professional.

Biotin supplements are available without a prescription in the following dosage forms:

Oral
- Capsules (U.S.)
- Tablets (U.S. and Canada)

Importance of Diet

Biotin is found in various foods, including liver, cauliflower, salmon, carrots, bananas, soy flour, cereals, and yeast. Biotin content of food is reduced by cooking and preserving.

Normal daily recommended intakes for biotin are generally defined as follows:
- Infants and children—
  Birth to 3 years of age: 10 to 20 micrograms (mcg).
  4 to 6 years: 25 mcg.
  7 to 10 years: 30 mcg.
- Adolescents and adults—30 to 100 mcg.

Side Effects of This Dietary Supplement

No side effects have been reported for biotin in amounts up to 10 milligrams a day. However, check with your health care professional if you notice any unusual effects while you are taking it.

Other Claimed Uses

Claims that biotin supplements are effective in the treatment of acne, eczema (a type of skin disorder), or hair loss have not been proven.

CALCIUM SUPPLEMENTS Systemic

Some commonly used brand names are:

In the U.S.—

Alka-Mints[1]
Amitone[1]
Calcarb 600[1]
Calci-Chew[1]
Calciday 667[1]
Calcilac[1]
Calci-Mix[1]
Calcium 600[1]
Calglycine[1]
Calphosan[7]
Cal-Plus[1]
Caltrate 600[1]
Caltrate Jr.[1]
Chooz[1]
Citracal[3]
Citracal Liquitabs[3]
Dicarbosil[1]
Gencalc 600[1]
Kalcinate[6]

Liquid-Cal[1]
Liquid Cal-600[1]
Maalox Antacid
  Caplets[1]
Mallamint[1]
Neo-Calglucon[4]
Nephro-Calci[1]
Os-Cal 500[1]
Os-Cal 500 Chewable[1]
Oysco[1]
Oysco 500 Chewable[1]
Oyst-Cal 500[1]
Oystercal 500[1]
Posture[11]
Rolaids Calcium Rich[1]
Titralac[1]
Tums[1]
Tums 500[1]
Tums E-X[1]

In Canada—

Apo-Cal[1]
Calciject[2]
Calcite 500[1]
Calcium-Sandoz[4]
Calcium-Sandoz Forte[9]
Calcium Stanley[5]
Calsan[1]

Caltrate 600[1]
Gramcal[9]
Nu-Cal[1]
Os-Cal[1]
Os-Cal Chewable[1]
Tums Extra Strength[1]
Tums Regular Strength[1]

Note: For quick reference, the following calcium supplements are numbered to match the corresponding brand names.

This information applies to the following:

1. Calcium Carbonate (KAL-see-um KAR-boh-nate)‡§
2. Calcium Chloride (KLOR-ide)‡§

3. Calcium Citrate (SIH-trayt)†‡
4. Calcium Glubionate (gloo-BY-oh-nate)§
5. Calcium Gluceptate and Calcium Gluconate (GLOO-coh-nate)*
6. Calcium Gluconate‡§
7. Calcium Glycerophosphate (gliss-er-o-FOS-fate) and Calcium Lactate (LAK-tate)†
8. Calcium Lactate‡§
9. Calcium Lactate-Gluconate and Calcium Carbonate*
10. Dibasic (dy-BAY-sic) Calcium Phosphate (FOS-fate)†‡
11. Tribasic (try-BAY-sic) Calcium Phosphate†

---

*Not commercially available in the U.S.

†Not commercially available in Canada.

‡Generic name product may also be available in the U.S.

§Generic name product may also be available in Canada.

#In Canada, calcium glubionate is known as calcium glucono-galacto gluconate.

Description

Calcium supplements are taken by individuals who are unable to get enough calcium in their regular diet or who have a need for more calcium. They are used to prevent or treat several conditions that may cause hypocalcemia (not enough calcium in the blood). The body needs calcium to make strong bones. Calcium is also needed for the heart, muscles, and nervous system to work properly.

The bones serve as a storage site for the body's calcium. They are continuously giving up calcium to the bloodstream and then replacing it as the body's need for calcium changes from day to day. When there is not enough calcium in the blood to be used by the heart and other organs, your body will take the needed calcium from the bones. When you eat foods rich in calcium, the calcium will be restored to the bones and the balance between your blood and bones will be maintained.

Pregnant women, nursing mothers, children, and adolescents may need more calcium than they normally get from eating calcium-rich foods. Adult women may take calcium supplements to help prevent a bone disease called osteoporosis. Other bone diseases in children and adults are also treated with calcium supplements.

Calcium and Osteoporosis

Bone is continually broken down and rebuilt, and calcium is necessary for the process of rebuilding. A lack of calcium causes a loss of calcium from the bone, resulting in osteoporosis. As men and women get older, their bodies build new bone at a slower rate. Because of a reduced amount of ovarian estrogen (a female hormone) at menopause, women's bodies begin to break down bone faster than it can be rebuilt. Therefore, osteoporosis is more common in older adults, especially in women.

Many studies have found that high intakes of calcium (through the diet or supplements or both) benefit bone quality in all age groups, possibly preventing osteoporosis. In particular, several studies have found that calcium supplements in amounts of 1000 to 1700 milligrams (mg) a day (alone and in combination with vitamin D or estrogen) have slowed bone loss in postmenopausal women. The evidence is strong enough that the Food and Drug Administration (FDA) allows food and supplement manufacturers to claim that calcium-rich products help prevent osteoporosis.

In a recent National Institutes of Health (NIH) conference on optimal calcium intake, the expert panel recommended that the daily intake for calcium be increased in all adults. In addition, the panel also reported that a large percentage of Americans do not get enough calcium in their diets. The preferred source of calcium, according to the panel, is through calcium-rich foods. However, calcium supplements are another way to meet optimal calcium intake.

From evidence available, it is fairly well established that increased calcium consumption is beneficial in reducing the risk and progression of osteoporosis.

The following studies looked at calcium intake and the prevention of osteoporosis in postmenopausal women: *New England Journal of Medicine*, 1992, Volume 327, pages 1637-

1642; *New England Journal of Medicine*, 1993, Volume 328, pages 460-464; and *Annals of Internal Medicine*, 1994, Volume 120, pages 97-103. Additional information on calcium can be found in the following publications: *Consumer Reports on Health*, February 1994, pages 13-15; *Nutrition Action Healthletter*, June 1994, pages 1, 5-9.

Availability

Injectable calcium is administered only by or under the supervision of your health care professional. Other forms of calcium are available without a prescription.

Calcium supplements are available in the following dosage forms:

Oral

Calcium Carbonate
- Capsules (U.S. and Canada)
- Oral suspension (U.S.)
- Tablets (U.S. and Canada)
- Chewable tablets (U.S. and Canada)

Calcium Citrate
- Tablets (U.S.)
- Tablets for solution (U.S.)

Calcium Glubionate
- Syrup (U.S. and Canada)

Calcium Gluceptate and Calcium Gluconate
- Oral solution (Canada)

Calcium Gluconate
- Tablets (U.S. and Canada)
- Chewable tablets (U.S.)

Calcium Lactate
- Tablets (U.S. and Canada)

Calcium Lactate-Gluconate and Calcium Carbonate
- Tablets for solution (Canada)

Dibasic Calcium Phosphate
- Tablets (U.S.)

Tribasic Calcium Phosphate
- Tablets (U.S.)

Parenteral

Calcium Chloride
- Injection (U.S. and Canada)

Calcium Glubionate
- Injection (Canada)

Calcium Gluceptate
- Injection (U.S.)

Calcium Gluconate
- Injection (U.S. and Canada)

Calcium Glycerophosphate and Calcium Lactate
- Injection (U.S.)

A calcium "salt" contains calcium along with another substance, such as carbonate or gluconate. Some calcium salts have more calcium (elemental calcium) than others. For example, the amount of calcium in calcium carbonate is greater than that in calcium gluconate. To give you an idea of how different calcium supplements vary in calcium content, the following chart explains how many tablets of each type of supplement will provide 1000 milligrams (mg) of elemental calcium. When you look for a calcium supplement, be sure the number of milligrams on the label refers to the amount of elemental calcium, and not to the strength of each tablet.

Calcium supplement	Strength of each tablet (mg)	Amount of elemental calcium per tablet (mg)	Number of tablets to provide 1000 mg of calcium
Calcium carbonate	625	250	4
	650	260	4
	750	300	4
	835	334	3
	1250	500	2
	1500	600	2
Calcium citrate	950	200	5
Calcium gluconate	500	45	22
	650	58	17
	1000	90	11
Calcium lactate	325	42	24
	650	84	12
Calcium phos-phate, dibasic	500	115	9
Calcium phos-phate, tribasic	800	304	4
	1600	608	2

Importance of Diet

Many nutritionists recommend that, if possible, people should get all the calcium they need from foods. However, some people may not be able to tolerate milk products because their bodies lack an enzyme called lactase, which helps the body digest milk. For such people, a calcium supplement is important.

Getting the proper amount of calcium in the

diet every day and participating in weight-bearing exercise (walking, dancing, bicycling, aerobics, jogging), especially during the early years of life (up to about 35 years of age) is most important in helping to build and maintain bones as dense as possible to prevent the development of osteoporosis in later life.

The following table includes some calcium-rich foods:

Food (amount)	Calcium (milligrams)
Nonfat dry milk, reconstituted (1 cup)	375
Lowfat, skim, or whole milk (1 cup)	290 to 300
Yogurt (1 cup)	275 to 400
Sardines with bones (3 ounces)	370
Ricotta cheese, part skim (½ cup)	340
Salmon, canned, with bones (3 ounces)	285
Cheese, Swiss (1 ounce)	272
Cheese, cheddar (1 ounce)	204
Cheese, American (1 ounce)	174
Cottage cheese, lowfat (1 cup)	154
Tofu (4 ounces)	154
Shrimp (1 cup)	147
Ice milk (¾ cup)	132

Vitamin D helps prevent calcium loss from your bones. It is sometimes called "the sunshine vitamin" because it is made in your skin when you are exposed to sunlight. If you get outside in the sunlight every day for 15 to 30 minutes, you should get all the vitamin D you need. However, in northern locations in winter, the sunlight may be too weak to make vitamin D in the skin. Vitamin D may also be obtained from your diet or from multivitamin preparations. Most milk is fortified with vitamin D.

Do not use bonemeal or dolomite as a source of calcium. The Food and Drug Administration has issued warnings that bonemeal and dolomite could be dangerous because these products may contain lead.

Normal daily recommended intakes in milligrams (mg) for calcium are generally defined as follows:

Persons	U.S. (mg)	Canada (mg)
Infants and children		
Birth to 3 years of age	400–800	250–550
4 to 6 years of age	800	600
7 to 10 years of age	800	700–1100
Adolescent and adult		
males	800–1200	800–1100
Adolescent and adult		
females	800–1200	700–1100
Pregnant females	1200	1200–1500
Breast-feeding females	1200	1200–1500

Before Using This Dietary Supplement

If you are taking this dietary supplement without a prescription, carefully read and follow any precautions on the label. For calcium supplements, the following should be considered:

Children—Injectable forms of calcium should

not be given to children because of the risk of irritation at the injection site.

Older adults—Some older people may need to take extra calcium or larger doses because they do not absorb calcium as well as younger people. Check with your health care professional if you have any questions about the amount of calcium you should be taking in each day.

Medicines or other dietary supplements—Although certain medicines or dietary supplements should not be used together at all, in other cases they may be used together even if an interaction might occur. In these cases, your health care professional may want to change the dose, or other precautions may be necessary. When you are taking calcium supplements, it is especially important that your health care professional know if you are taking any of the following:

- Calcium-containing medicines, other—Taking excess calcium may cause too much calcium in the blood or urine and lead to medical problems
- Cellulose sodium phosphate (e.g., Calcibind)—Use with calcium supplements may decrease the effects of cellulose sodium phosphate
- Digitalis glycosides (heart medicine)—Use with calcium supplements by injection may increase the chance of irregular heartbeat
- Etidronate (e.g., Didronel)—Use with calcium supplements may decrease the effects of eti-

dronate; etidronate should not be taken within 2 hours of calcium supplements

- Gallium nitrate (e.g., Ganite)—Use with calcium supplements may cause gallium nitrate to not work properly
- Magnesium sulfate (for injection)—Use with calcium supplements may cause either to be less effective
- Phenytoin (e.g., Dilantin)—Use with calcium supplements may decrease the effects of both; calcium supplements should not be taken within 1 to 3 hours of phenytoin
- Tetracyclines (medicine for infection) taken by mouth—Use with calcium supplements may decrease the effects of tetracycline; calcium supplements should not be taken within 1 to 3 hours of tetracyclines

Other medical problems—The presence of other medical problems may affect the use of calcium supplements. Make sure you tell your health care professional if you have any other medical problems, especially:

- Diarrhea or
- Stomach or intestinal problems—Extra calcium or specific calcium preparations may be necessary in these conditions
- Heart disease—Calcium by injection may increase the chance of irregular heartbeat
- Hypercalcemia (too much calcium in the blood) or
- Hypercalciuria (too much calcium in the urine)—Calcium supplements may make these conditions worse
- Hyperparathyroidism or
- Sarcoidosis—Calcium supplements may in-

crease the chance of hypercalcemia (too much calcium in the blood)

- Hypoparathyroidism—Use of calcium phosphate may cause high blood levels of phosphorus which could increase the chance of side effects
- Kidney disease or stones—Too much calcium may increase the chance of kidney stones

---

Proper Use of This Dietary Supplement

Drink a full glass (8 ounces) of water or juice when taking a calcium supplement.

This dietary supplement is best taken 1 to 1½ hours after meals, unless otherwise directed by your health care professional. However, patients with a condition known as achlorhydria may not absorb calcium supplements on an empty stomach and should take them with meals.

For individuals taking *the chewable tablet form* of this dietary supplement:

- Chew the tablets completely before swallowing.

For individuals taking *the syrup form* of this dietary supplement:

- Take the syrup before meals. This will allow the dietary supplement to work faster.
- Mix in water or fruit juice for infants or children.

Precautions While Using This Dietary Supplement

If this dietary supplement has been ordered for you by your doctor and you will be taking it in large doses or for a long time, your doctor should check your progress at regular visits. This is to make sure the calcium is working properly and does not cause unwanted effects.

Do not take calcium supplements within 1 to 2 hours of taking other medicine by mouth. To do so may keep the other medicine from working properly.

Unless you are otherwise directed by your health care professional, to make sure that calcium is used properly by your body:

- *Do not take other medicines or dietary supplements containing large amounts of calcium, phosphates, magnesium, or vitamin D unless your health care professional has told you to do so or approved.*
- *Do not take calcium supplements within 1 to 2 hours of eating large amounts of fiber-containing foods, such as bran and whole-grain cereals or breads, especially if you are being treated for hypocalcemia (not enough calcium in your blood).*
- *Do not drink large amounts of alcohol or caffeine-containing beverages (usually more than 8 cups of coffee a day), or use tobacco.*

Some calcium carbonate tablets have been shown to break up too slowly in the stomach to be properly absorbed into the body. If the calcium carbonate tablets you purchase are not specifically labeled as being "USP," check with your pharmacist. He or she may be able to help you determine which tablets are best.

Side Effects of This Dietary Supplement

Along with its needed effects, a dietary supplement may cause some unwanted effects. Although the following side effects occur very rarely when the calcium supplement is taken as recommended, they may be more likely to occur if:

- It is taken in large doses.
- It is taken for a long time.
- It is taken by patients with kidney disease.

Check with your health care professional as soon as possible if any of the following side effects occur:

More common (for injection form only)

>   Dizziness; flushing and/or sensation of warmth or heat; irregular heartbeat; nausea or vomiting; skin redness, rash, pain, or burning at injection site; sweating; tingling sensation

Rare

>   Drowsiness; difficult or painful urination; nausea or vomiting (continuing); weakness

Early signs of overdose

>   Constipation (severe); dryness of mouth; headache (continuing); increased thirst; ir-

ritability; loss of appetite; mental depression; metallic taste; unusual tiredness or weakness

Late signs of overdose

Confusion; drowsiness (severe); high blood pressure; increased sensitivity of eyes or skin to light; irregular, fast, or slow heartbeat; unusually large amount of urine or increased frequency of urination

Other side effects not listed above may also occur in some individuals. If you notice any other effects, check with your health care professional.

Other Claimed Uses

Calcium and Blood Pressure

Claimed use: Some people think that increasing calcium intake is useful in maintaining lower blood pressure.

Possible action: Calcium is involved in many body functions (e.g., bone strength, muscle movement). It is believed that calcium lowers blood pressure by relaxing the blood vessels. This allows the blood to move more easily throughout your body, thus decreasing the workload of your heart.

Current findings: Some studies have found that certain patients who took 1000 to 1500 milligrams (mg) of calcium a day had a slight lowering of blood pressure, compared to patients who received a pill that did not contain calcium (placebo). These studies found that taking calcium supplements for four weeks or longer lowered blood pressure by 2 to 8 points. Other studies have found that calcium supplements may lower blood pressure or prevent the high blood pressure that may occur in some women during pregnancy. The pregnant women in the studies took 1000 to 2000 mg of calcium a day during their last 6 months of pregnancy.

Role of diet: Many studies have found that people who get enough calcium in their diet have lower blood pressure than those who do not.

Conclusion: It appears that adequate calcium in the diet is associated with lower blood pressure. Some studies show that calcium supplements may help to maintain a lower blood pressure. However, people with high blood pressure should discuss the role of calcium with their health care professional.

Additional reading: The following review article looked at calcium supplements in the treatment of high blood pressure: *Drugs*, 1990, Volume 39, pages 7-18. The following study looked at calcium supplements in the prevention of high blood pressure in pregnant women: *New England Journal of Medicine*, 1991, Volume 325, pages 1399-1405. More information on calcium supplements can be found in *Consumer Reports on Health*, February 1994, Volume 6, pages 13-15.

CHROMIUM SUPPLEMENTS Systemic

This information applies to the following:

1. Chromic Chloride (KROME-ik KLOR-ide)‡
2. Chromium (KROH-mee-um)‡§

---

‡Generic name product may also be available in the U.S.

§Generic name product may also be available in Canada.

Description

Chromium supplements are used to prevent or treat chromium deficiency.

The body needs chromium for normal growth and health. For patients who are unable to get enough chromium in their regular diet or who have a need for more chromium, chromium supplements may be necessary. They are generally taken by mouth but some patients may have to receive them by injection. Chromium helps your body use sugar properly. It is also needed for metabolism of proteins and fats.

Lack of chromium may lead to nerve problems and may decrease the body's ability to use sugar properly.

Injectable chromium is administered only by or under the supervision of your health care professional. Other forms of chromium are available without a prescription.

Chromium supplements are available in the following dosage forms:

Oral

Chromium
  • Capsules (U.S.)
  • Tablets (U.S. and Canada)

Parenteral

Chromic Chloride
  • Injection (U.S. and Canada)

Importance of Diet

Chromium is found in various foods, including brewer's yeast, calf liver, American cheese, and wheat germ.

Normal daily recommended intakes for chromium are generally defined as follows:

  • Infants and children—
    Birth to 3 years of age: 10–80 micrograms (mcg).
    4 to 6 years of age: 30–120 mcg.
    7 to 10 years of age: 50–200 mcg.
  • Adolescents and adults—50–200 mcg.

Before Using This Dietary Supplement

If you are taking this dietary supplement without a prescription, carefully read and follow any precautions on the label. For chromium, the following should be considered:

Other medical problems—The presence of other medical problems may affect the use of

chromium. Make sure you tell your health care professional if you have any other medical problems, especially:

- Diabetes mellitus (sugar diabetes)—Taking chromium supplements when you have a chromium deficiency may cause a change in the amount of insulin you need

Side Effects of This Dietary Supplement

No side effects have been reported for chromium. However, check with your health care professional if you notice any unusual effects while you are taking it.

Other Claimed Uses

There is not enough evidence to show that chromium supplements may improve the way your body uses sugar (glucose tolerance) if you are not deficient in chromium.

Chromium and Exercise Physiology

Claimed use: Some people think that taking chromium supplements (particularly chromium picolinate) will decrease body sugar and fat and increase muscle size and strength.

Possible action: You need chromium in your diet to help your body use its natural insulin. Insulin helps your body break down carbohydrates and fats.

Current findings: There have been two studies in which groups of athletes were given chromium supplements. In one study, 38 football players were given 200 micrograms (mcg) of chromium daily for 9 weeks. The researchers found that chromium supplements did not cause changes in body fat, body size, or body strength. Another study involved 59 students at the beginning of a weight training program. Half of the subjects received 200 mcg of chromium a day for 12 weeks and the other half received a pill that did not contain chromium (placebo). The study found that women who received chromium supplements gained more weight than either the women who received the placebo or the men who received chromium supplements or placebo. Body size and strength were not affected in either group.

Conclusion: Chromium supplements are useful only when a chromium deficiency is present. Studies performed to date provide little evidence that using chromium supplements decreases body fat and/or increases muscle size and strength.

Additional reading: The two studies mentioned above can be found in the *International Journal of Sports Nutrition,* 1994, Volume 4, pages 142-153 and *International Journal of Sports Nutrition,* 1992, Volume 2, pages 343-345.

COPPER
SUPPLEMENTS Systemic

A commonly used brand name is:

In the U.S.—
    Cupri-Pak[2]

Note: For quick reference, the following copper supplements are numbered to match the corresponding brand names.

This information applies to the following:

1. Copper Gluconate (KOP-er GLOO-coh-nate)‡
2. Cupric Sulfate (KYOO-prik SUL-fate)†‡

---

†Not commercially available in Canada.
‡Generic name product may also be available in the U.S.

Description

Copper supplements are used to prevent or treat copper deficiency.

The body needs copper for normal growth and health. For patients who are unable to get enough copper in their regular diet or who have a need for more copper, copper supplements may be necessary. They are generally taken by mouth but some patients may have to receive them by injection. Copper is needed to help your body use iron. It is also important for nerve function, bone growth, and to help your body use sugar.

Lack of copper may lead to anemia and osteoporosis (weak bones).

Some conditions may increase your need for copper. These include:

- Burns
- Diarrhea
- Intestinal diseases
- Kidney disease
- Pancreas disease
- Stomach removal
- Stress, continuing

In addition, premature infants may need additional copper.

Increased need for copper should be determined by your health care professional.

Injectable copper is administered only by or under the supervision of your health care professional. Another form of copper is available without a prescription.

Copper supplements are available in the following dosage forms:

Oral

Copper Gluconate
- Tablets (U.S.)

Parenteral

Cupric Sulfate
- Injection (U.S.)

Importance of Diet

Copper is found in various foods, including organ meats (especially liver), seafoods, beans, nuts, and whole-grains. Additional copper can come from drinking water from copper pipes, using copper cookware, and eating farm products sprayed with copper-containing chemicals. Copper may be decreased in foods that have high acid content and are stored in tin cans for a long time.

Normal daily recommended intakes are generally defined as follows:

- Infants and children—
  Birth to 3 years of age: 0.4 to 1 milligrams (mg) per day.
  4 to 6 years of age: 1 to 1.5 mg per day.
  7 to 10 years of age: 1 to 2 mg per day.
- Adolescent and adult males—1.5 to 2.5 mg per day.
- Adolescent and adult females—1.5 to 3 mg per day.

Before Using This Dietary Supplement

If you are taking this dietary supplement without a prescription, carefully read and follow any precautions on the label. For copper supplements, the following should be considered:

Medicines or other dietary supplements— Although certain medicines or dietary supplements should not be used together at all, in other cases they may be used together even if an interaction might occur. In these cases, your health care professional may want to change the dose, or other precautions may be necessary. When you are taking copper supplements, it is especially important that your health care professional know if you are taking any of the following:

- Penicillamine or
- Trientine or
- Zinc supplements (taken by mouth)—Use with copper supplements may decrease the amount of copper that gets into the body; copper supplements should be taken at least 2 hours after penicillamine, trientine, or zinc supplements

Other medical problems—The presence of other medical problems may affect the use of copper supplements. Make sure you tell your health care professional if you have any other medical problems, especially:

- Wilson's disease (too much copper in the body)—Copper supplements may make this condition worse
- Biliary disease or
- Liver disease—Taking copper supplements may cause high blood levels of copper, and dosage for copper may have to be changed

---

Precautions While Using This Dietary Supplement

Do not take copper supplements and zinc supplements at the same time. It is best to take your copper supplement 2 hours after zinc supplements, to get the full benefit of each.

Side Effects of This Dietary Supplement

Along with its needed effects, a dietary supplement may cause some unwanted effects. Although copper supplements have not been reported to cause any side effects, *check with your health care professional immediately* if any of the following side effects occur as a result of an overdose:

Symptoms of overdose

Black or bloody vomit; blood in urine; coma; diarrhea; dizziness or fainting; headache (severe or continuing); heartburn; loss of appetite; lower back pain; metallic taste; nausea (severe or continuing); pain or burning while urinating; vomiting; yellow eyes or skin

Other side effects not listed above may also occur in some individuals. If you notice any other effects, check with your health care professional.

Other Claimed Uses

Claims that copper supplements are effective in the treatment of arthritis or skin conditions have not been proven. Use of copper supplements to cause vomiting has caused death and should be avoided.

ENTERAL NUTRITION FORMULAS   Systemic

Some commonly used brand names are:

In the U.S.—

Accupep HPF[6]
Alitraq[6]
Amin-Aid[2]
Attain[7]
Carnation Instant
  Breakfast[4]
Carnation Instant
  Breakfast No Sugar
  Added[4]
Casec[5]
CitriSource[7]
Citrotein[7]
Compleat Modified[1]
Compleat Regular[1]
Comply[7]
Criticare HN[6]
Elementra[5]
Ensure[7]
Ensure with Fiber[3]
Ensure HN[7]
Ensure Plus[7]
Ensure Plus HN[7]
Entrition Half-Strength[7]
Entrition HN[7]
Fiberlan[3]
Fibersource[3]
Fibersource HN[3]
Glucerna[2]
Great Shake[4]
Hepatic-Aid II[2]
Immun-Aid[2]
Impact[2]
Impact with Fiber[2,3]
Introlan[7]
Introlite[7]

Isocal[7]
Isocal HCN[7]
Isocal HN[7]
Isolan[7]
Isosource[7]
Isosource HN[7]
Isotein HN[7]
Jevity[3]
Lipisorb[2]
Lonalac[4]
Magnacal[7]
MCT Oil[5]
Menu Magic Instant
  Breakfast[4]
Menu Magic Milk
  Shake[4]
Meritene[4]
Microlipid[5]
Moducal[5]
Nepro[2]
Nutren 1.0[7]
Nutren 1.5[7]
Nutren 2.0[7]
Nutren 1.0 with Fiber[3]
NutriHep[2]
Nutrilan Flavored
  Supplements[7]
NutriSource[3]
NutriSource HN[3]
NutriVent[2]
Osmolite[7]
Osmolite HN[7]
Pediasure[7]
Pediasure with Fiber[3]
Peptamen[6]

In the U.S. (cont'd)—

Perative[2]
Polycose[5]
Pre-Attain[7]
Precision HN[7]
Precision Isotonic Diet[7]
Precision Low Residue[7]
Profiber[3]
ProMod[5]
Promote[7]
Propac[5]
Protain XL[2]
Pulmocare[2]
Reabilan[6]
Reabilan HN[6]
Replete[7]
Replete with Fiber[3]
Resource[7]
Resource Plus[7]
Stresstein[2]
Sumacal[5]

Suplena[2]
Sustacal[7]
Sustacal 8.8[7]
Sustacal with Fiber[3]
Sustacal HC[7]
Sustagen[4]
Tasty Shake[4]
Tolerex[6]
TraumaCal[2]
Traum-Aid HBC[2]
Travasorb Hepatic Diet[2]
Travasorb HN[6]
Travasorb Renal Diet[2]
Travasorb STD[6]
TwoCal HN[7]
Ultracal[3]
Ultralan[7]
Vital High Nitrogen[6]
Vitaneed[1]
Vivonex T.E.N.[6]

In Canada—

CitriSource[7]
Citrotein[2]
Compleat Modified[1]
Enercal[7]
Ensure[7]
Ensure with Fiber[3]
Ensure High Protein[7]
Ensure Plus[7]
Glucerna[2]
Impact[2]
Isosource[7]
Isosource HN[7]
Jevity[3]
MCT Oil[5]
Meritene[4]

Nepro[2]
NutriSource[3]
NutriSource HN[3]
Osmolite HN[7]
Pediasure[7]
Polycose[5]
ProMod[5]
Pulmocare[2]
Resource[7]
Resource Plus[7]
Suplena[2]
Sustagen[4]
Tolerex[6]
Vital High Nitrogen[6]
Vivonex T.E.N.[6]

Note: For quick reference, the following enteral nutrition formulas are numbered to match the corresponding brand names.

This information applies to the following enteral nutrition formulas:

1. Enteral nutrition formulas, blenderized
2. Enteral nutrition formulas, disease-specific
3. Enteral nutrition formulas, fiber-containing
4. Enteral nutrition formulas, milk-based
5. Enteral nutrition formulas, modular
6. Enteral nutrition formulas, monomeric (elemental)
7. Enteral nutrition formulas, polymeric

Description

Enteral nutrition formulas are used as nutritional replacements for patients who are unable to get enough nutrients in their diet. These formulas are taken by mouth or through a feeding tube and are used by the body for energy and to form substances needed for normal body functions.

Patients with the following conditions may be more likely to need enteral feedings:

- Acquired immune deficiency syndrome (AIDS)
- Burns
- Cancer
- Infections, prolonged
- Kidney problems
- Liver problems
- Lung problems
- Pancreas problems
- Stomach problems
- Surgery
- Trauma
- Vomiting, prolonged

Enteral nutrition formulas are available without a prescription. However, they should only be used under medical supervision.

The benefits of enteral formulas in healthy people have not been proven.

Enteral nutrition formulas are available in the following dosage forms:

Oral

Blenderized Enteral Nutrition
- Oral solution (U.S. and Canada)

Disease-specific Enteral Nutrition
- Oral solution (U.S. and Canada)
- Powder for solution (U.S. and Canada)

Fiber-containing Enteral Nutrition
- Oral solution (U.S. and Canada)

Milk-based Enteral Nutrition
- Oral solution (U.S.)
- Powder for solution (U.S. and Canada)

Modular Enteral Nutrition
- Oil (U.S. and Canada)
- Oral solution (U.S. and Canada)
- Oral powder (U.S. and Canada)

Monomeric Enteral Nutrition
- Oral solution (U.S. and Canada)
- Powder for solution (U.S.)

Polymeric Enteral Nutrition
- Oral solution (U.S. and Canada)
- Powder for solution (U.S.)

Before Using This Enteral Nutrition Formula

If you are taking any of these enteral nutrition formulas without a prescription, carefully read and follow any precautions on the label.

For enteral nutrition formulas, the following should be considered:

Children—Caution should be used when giving enteral feedings to children less than one year of age. Very young children may not be able to eliminate the feeding from the body. Although there is no specific information about the use of enteral feedings in older children, it is not expected to cause different side effects or problems in these children than it does in adults.

Older adults—Older adults may be at risk of developing problems related to the use of a nasogastric tube (tube going through the nose into the stomach), such as aspiration (sucking fluid into the lungs) or removing the nasogastric tube. The enteral feeding itself has not been shown to cause different side effects or problems in older people than it does in younger adults.

Other medical problems—The presence of other medical problems may affect the use of enteral feedings. Make sure you tell your health care professional if you have any other medical problems, especially:

- Breathing problems or
- Dehydration or
- Diabetes mellitus (sugar diabetes) or
- Diarrhea or
- Heart problems or
- Hyperglycemia (high levels of sugar in the blood) or
- Hyperlipidemia or
- Lactose intolerance or

- Liver problems or
- Pancreas problems—Enteral feedings may make these conditions worse; your health care professional may recommend a special formula for your condition
- Intestine problems or
- Stomach problems—These problems may prevent enteral formulas from being absorbed properly
- Kidney problems—Higher blood levels of certain ingredients of the enteral feeding may result, and a smaller amount of enteral feeding may be needed
- Malnutrition, severe—Heart and nerve problems have been reported when feeding a patient who is severely malnourished; enteral formula may need to be used in smaller amounts

---

Proper Use of This Enteral Nutrition Formula

Your enteral feeding may be given by mouth or by a feeding tube. Use the amount recommended by your health care professional.

For patients taking the *oral liquid* form of enteral nutrition:

- This preparation is in ready-to-use form. No dilution is needed unless directed by your health care professional.
- Shake the preparation well before opening. Refrigerate after opening, out of the reach of children. Most formulas can be

kept in the refrigerator for 1 to 2 days. Check the label of your product.

For patients using the *powder* form of this preparation:

• For mixing or other use, follow carefully the instructions on the package.

• Any unused solution should be kept in the refrigerator, out of the reach of children. Most formulas can be kept in the refrigerator for 1 to 2 days. Check the label of your product.

Precautions While Using This Enteral Nutrition Formula

Enteral feedings must be handled properly to protect them from bacteria. Enteral feedings should be used for no more than 12 hours at room temperature and then should be discarded.

If you are taking your enteral feeding through a tube, enteral formulas that are too thick may clog the feeding tube. If this happens, check with your health care professional.

Side Effects of This Enteral Nutrition Formula

Some problems may result from improper use of an enteral formula or use of the incorrect formula in your condition. Check with your health care professional if any of the following problems occur:

More common

Confusion; convulsions (seizures); decrease in urine volume; dryness of mouth; frequent urination; increased thirst; irregular heartbeat; mood or mental changes; muscle cramps or pain; numbness or tingling in hands, feet, or lips; respiratory distress, shortness of breath or difficulty breathing; unexplained nervousness; unusual tiredness or weakness; weakness or heaviness of legs; weak pulse

Other problems may occur that usually do not need medical attention. They may go away during treatment as your body adjusts to the enteral nutrition formula. However, check with your health care professional if any of the following side effects continue or are bothersome:

More common

Constipation; diarrhea; nausea or vomiting

Other side effects not listed above may also occur in some patients. If you notice any other effects, check with your health care professional.

FOLIC ACID (Vitamin B₉)
Systemic

Some commonly used brand names are:

In the U.S.—
Folvite
Generic name product may also be available.

In Canada—
Apo-Folic   Novo-Folacid
Folvite
Generic name product may also be available.

Another commonly used name is Vitamin B_9.

Description

Vitamins (VYE-ta-mins) are compounds that you *must* have for growth and health. They are needed in small amounts only and are usually available in the foods that you eat. Folic (FOE-lik) acid (vitamin B_9) is necessary for strong blood.

Lack of folic acid may lead to anemia (weak blood). Your health care professional may treat this by prescribing folic acid for you.

Some conditions may increase your need for folic acid. These include:

- Alcoholism
- Anemia, hemolytic
- Diarrhea (continuing)
- Fever (prolonged)
- Hemodialysis
- Illness (prolonged)

- Intestinal diseases
- Liver disease
- Stress (continuing)
- Surgical removal of stomach

In addition, infants smaller than normal, breast-fed infants, or those receiving unfortified formulas (such as evaporated milk or goat's milk) may need additional folic acid.

Increased need for folic acid should be determined by your health care professional.

Some studies have found that 400 micrograms of folic acid consumed by women before they become pregnant and during early pregnancy may reduce the chances of certain birth defects (neural tube defects).

Injectable folic acid is administered only by or under the supervision of your health care professional. Some strengths of oral folic acid are available only with a prescription. Others are available without a prescription.

Folic acid is available in the following dosage forms:

Oral
- Tablets (U.S. and Canada)

Parenteral
- Injection (U.S. and Canada)

Importance of Diet

Folic acid is found in various foods, including vegetables, especially green vegetables; potatoes; cereal and cereal products; fruits; and organ meats (for example, liver or kidney). It is best to eat fresh fruits and vegetables whenever possible since they contain the most vitamins. Food processing may destroy some of the vitamins. For example, heat may reduce the amount of folic acid in foods.

Normal daily recommended intakes in micrograms (mcg) for folic acid are generally defined as follows:

Persons	U.S. (mcg)	Canada (mcg)
Infants and children		
Birth to 3 years of age	25–50	50–80
4 to 6 years of age	75	90
7 to 10 years of age	100	125–180
Adolescent and adult males	150–200	150–220
Adolescent and adult females	150–180	145–190
Pregnant females	400	445–475
Breast-feeding females	260–280	245–275

Before Using This Dietary Supplement
In deciding to use this dietary supplement, the risks of taking it must be weighed against the good it will do. This is a decision you and your health care professional will make. For folic acid, the following should be considered:

Pregnancy—Your health care professional may recommend that you consume folic acid from foods or as a supplement or as part of a multivitamin supplement before you become pregnant and during early pregnancy. It is recommended that you receive 400 micrograms (mcg) of folic acid a day. Folic acid may reduce the chances of your baby being born with certain types of birth defects (neural tube defects).

Other medical problems—The presence of other medical problems may affect the use of folic acid. Make sure you tell your health care professional if you have any other medical problems, especially:

- Pernicious anemia (a type of blood problem)—Taking folic acid while you have pernicious anemia may cause serious side effects. You should be sure that you do not have pernicious anemia before beginning folic acid supplementation

---

Side Effects of This Dietary Supplement

Along with its needed effects, a dietary supplement may cause some unwanted effects. Although folic acid does not usually cause any side effects, check with your health care professional as soon as possible if any of the following side effects occur:

Rare

Fever; reddened skin; shortness of breath; skin rash or itching; tightness in chest; troubled breathing; wheezing

Other side effects not listed above may also occur in some individuals. If you notice any other effects, check with your health care professional.

Other Claimed Uses

Claims that folic acid and other B vitamins are effective for preventing mental problems have not been proven. Many of these treatments involve large and expensive amounts of vitamins.

IRON SUPPLEMENTS -Systemic

Some commonly used brand names are:

In the U.S.—

Femiron[1]	Ferra-TD[3]
Feosol[3]	Fumasorb[1]
Feostat[1]	Fumerin[1]
Feostat Drops[1]	Hemocyte[1]
Feratab[3]	Hytinic[5]
Fer-Gen-Sol[3]	InFeD[4]
Fergon[2]	Ircon[1]
Fer-In-Sol Capsules[3]	Mol-Iron[3]
Fer-In-Sol Drops[3]	Nephro-Fer[1]
Fer-In-Sol Syrup[3]	Niferex[5]
Fer-Iron Drops[3]	Niferex-150[5]
Fero-Gradumet[3]	Nu-Iron[5]
Ferospace[3]	Nu-Iron 150[5]
Ferralet[2]	Simron[2]
Ferralet Slow Release[2]	Slow Fe[3]
Ferralyn Lanacaps[3]	Span-FF[1]

In Canada

Apo-Ferrous Gluconate[2]	Neo-Fer[1]
Apo-Ferrous Sulfate[3]	Novoferrogluc[2]
Fer-In-Sol Drops[3]	Novoferrosulfa[3]
Fer-In-Sol Syrup[3]	Novofumar[1]
Fero-Grad[3]	Palafer[1]
Fertinic[2]	PMS Ferrous Sulfate[3]
Jectofer[6]	Slow Fe[3]

Note: For quick reference, the following iron supplements are numbered to match the corresponding brand names.

This information applies to the following:

1. Ferrous Fumarate (FER-us FYOO-ma-rate)‡
2. Ferrous Gluconate (FER-us GLOO-koe-nate)‡§
3. Ferrous Sulfate (FER-us SUL-fate)‡§
4. Iron Dextran (DEX-tran)
5. Iron-Polysaccharide (pol-i-SAK-a-ride)†
6. Iron Sorbitol (SOR-bi-tole)*

*Not commercially available in the U.S.

†Not commercially available in Canada.

‡Generic name product may also be available in the U.S.

§Generic name product may also be available in Canada.

Description

Iron is a mineral that the body needs to produce red blood cells. When the body does not get enough iron, it cannot produce the number of normal red blood cells needed to keep you in good health. This condition is called iron deficiency (iron shortage) or iron deficiency anemia.

Although many people in the U.S. get enough iron from their diet, some must take additional amounts to meet their needs. For example, iron is sometimes lost with slow or small amounts of bleeding in the body that you would not be aware of and which can only be detected by your health care professional. Your health care professional can determine if you have an iron deficiency, what is causing the deficiency, and if an iron supplement is necessary.

Lack of iron may lead to unusual tiredness, shortness of breath, a decrease in physical performance and learning problems in children and adults, and may increase your chance of getting an infection.

Some conditions may increase your need for iron. These include:

- Bleeding problems
- Burns
- Hemodialysis
- Intestinal diseases
- Stomach problems
- Stomach removal

In addition, infants, especially those receiving breast milk or low-iron formulas, may need additional iron.

Increased need for iron should be determined by your health care professional.

Injectable iron is administered only by or under the supervision of your health care professional. Other forms of iron are available without a prescription; however, your health care professional may have special instructions on the proper use and dose for your condition.

Iron supplements are available in the following dosage forms:

Oral

Ferrous Fumarate
- Capsules (Canada)
- Extended-release capsules (U.S.)
- Solution (U.S.)
- Suspension (U.S. and Canada)
- Tablets (U.S. and Canada)
- Chewable tablets (U.S.)

Ferrous Gluconate
- Capsules (U.S.)
- Elixir (U.S.)
- Syrup (Canada)

- Tablets (U.S. and Canada)
- Extended-release tablets (U.S.)

Ferrous Sulfate
- Capsules (U.S.)
- Extended-release capsules (U.S.)
- Elixir (U.S.)
- Solution (U.S. and Canada)
- Tablets (U.S. and Canada)
- Enteric-coated tablets (U.S. and Canada)
- Extended-release tablets (U.S. and Canada)

Iron-Polysaccharide
- Capsules (U.S.)
- Elixir (U.S.)
- Tablets (U.S.)

Parenteral

Iron Dextran
- Injection (U.S.)

Iron Sorbitol
- Injection (Canada)

Importance of Diet

Iron is found in the diet in two forms—heme iron, which is well absorbed, and nonheme iron, which is poorly absorbed. The best dietary source of absorbable (heme) iron is lean red meat. Chicken, turkey, and fish are also sources of iron, but they contain less than red meat. Cereals, beans, and some vegetables contain poorly absorbed (non-heme) iron. Foods rich in vitamin C (e.g., citrus fruits and fresh vegetables) eaten with small amounts of heme iron–containing foods, such as meat, may increase the amount of nonheme iron absorbed from cereals, beans, and other vegetables. Some foods (e.g., milk, eggs, spinach, fiber-containing coffee, tea) may decrease the amount of nonheme iron absorbed from foods. Additional iron may be added to food from cooking in iron pots.

Normal daily recommended intakes for iron are generally defined as follows (Note that the recommended intakes are expressed as an actual amount of iron, which is referred to as "elemental" iron. The drug form [e.g., ferrous fumarate, ferrous gluconate, ferrous sulfate] has a different strength):

Persons	U.S. (mg)	Canada (mg)
Infants and children		
Birth to 3 years of age	6–10	0.3–6
4 to 6 years of age	10	8
7 to 10 years of age	10	8–10
Adolescent and adult males	10–12	8–10
Adolescent and adult females	10–15	8–13
Pregnant females	30	23
Breast-feeding females	15	8–13

Before Using This Dietary Supplement

If you are taking this dietary supplement without a prescription, carefully read and follow any precautions on the label. For iron supplements, the following should be considered:

Pregnancy—During the first 3 months of pregnancy, a proper diet usually provides enough iron. However, during the last 6 months, in order to meet the increased needs of the developing baby, an iron supplement may be recommended by your health care professional.

Children—Iron supplements, when prescribed by your health care professional, are not expected to cause different side effects in children than they do in adults. However, it is important to follow the directions carefully, since iron overdose in children is especially dangerous.

Older adults—Elderly people sometimes do not absorb iron as easily as younger adults and may need a larger dose.

Medicines or other dietary supplements— Although certain medicines or dietary supplements should not be used together at all, in other cases they may be used together even if an interaction might occur. In these cases, your health care professional may want to change the dose, or other precautions may be necessary. When you are taking iron supplements, it is especially important that your health care professional know if you are taking any of the following:

- Acetohydroxamic acid (e.g., Lithostat)—Use with iron supplements may cause either medicine to be less effective
- Antacids—Use with iron supplements may make the iron supplements less effective; iron supplements should be taken 1 or 2 hours before or after antacids

- Dimercaprol—Iron supplements and dimercaprol may combine in the body to form a harmful chemical
- Etidronate or
- Fluoroquinolones (e.g., ciprofloxacin, enoxacin, lomefloxacin, norfloxacin, ofloxacin) or
- Tetracyclines (taken by mouth) (medicine for infection)—Use with iron supplements may make these medicines less effective; iron supplements should be taken 2 hours before or after these medicines

Other medical problems—The presence of other medical problems may affect the use of iron supplements. Make sure you tell your health care professional if you have any other medical problems, especially:

- Alcohol abuse (or history of) or
- Kidney infection or
- Liver disease or
- Porphyria cutaneous tarda—Higher blood levels of the iron supplement may occur, which may increase the chance of side effects
- Arthritis (rheumatoid) or
- Asthma or allergies or
- Heart disease—The injected form of iron may make these conditions worse
- Colitis or other intestinal problems or
- Iron overload conditions (e.g., hemochromatosis, hemosiderosis) or
- Stomach ulcer—Iron supplements may make these conditions worse

Proper Use of This Dietary Supplement

After you start using this dietary supplement, continue to return to your health care profes-

sional to see if you are benefiting from the
iron. Some blood tests may be necessary for
this.

Iron is best absorbed when taken on an empty
stomach, with water or fruit juice (adults: full
glass or 8 ounces; children: ½ glass or 4
ounces), about 1 hour before or 2 hours after
meals. However, to lessen the possibility of
stomach upset, iron may be taken with food
or immediately after meals.

For safe and effective use of iron supplements:

- Follow your health care professional's instructions if this dietary supplement
  was prescribed.
- Follow the manufacturer's package directions if you are treating yourself. If you
  think you still need iron after taking it
  for 1 or 2 months, check with your health
  care professional.

Liquid forms of iron supplement tend to stain the
teeth. To prevent, reduce, or remove these
stains:

- Mix each dose in water, fruit juice, or
  tomato juice. You may use a drinking
  tube or straw to help keep the iron supplement from getting on the teeth.
- When doses of liquid iron supplement
  are to be given by dropper, the dose may
  be placed well back on the tongue and
  followed with water or juice.
- Iron stains on teeth can usually be re-

moved by brushing with baking soda (sodium bicarbonate) or medicinal peroxide (hydrogen peroxide 3%).

Precautions While Using This Dietary Supplement

When iron is combined with certain foods it may lose much of its value. If you are taking iron, the following foods should be avoided or taken only in very small amounts for at least 1 hour before or 2 hours after you take iron:

Cheese and yogurt
Eggs
Milk
Spinach
Tea or coffee
Whole-grain breads and cereals and bran

Do not take iron supplements and antacids or calcium supplements at the same time. It is best to space doses of these 2 products 1 to 2 hours apart, to get the full benefit from each medicine or dietary supplement.

If you are taking iron supplement *without a prescription:*

- Do not take iron supplements by mouth if you are receiving iron injections. To do so may result in iron poisoning.

- Do not regularly take large amounts of iron for longer than 6 months without checking with your health care professional. People differ in their need for iron, and those with certain medical conditions can gradually become poisoned by taking too much iron over a period of time.

If you have been taking a long-acting or coated iron tablet and your stools have *not* become black, check with your health care professional. The tablets may not be breaking down properly in your stomach, and you may not be receiving enough iron.

It is important to keep iron preparations out of the reach of children. Keep a 1-ounce bottle of *syrup* of ipecac available at home to be taken in case of an iron overdose emergency when a health care professional, poison control center, or emergency room orders its use.

If you think you or anyone else has taken an overdose of iron:

- *Immediate medical attention is very important.*
- *Call your health care professional, a poison control center, or the nearest hospital emergency room at once. Always keep these phone numbers readily available.*
- *Follow any instructions given to you. If syrup of ipecac has been ordered and given, do not delay going to the emergency room while waiting for the ipecac syrup to empty the stomach, since it may require 20 to 30 minutes to show results.*
- *Go to the emergency room without delay.*
- *Take the container of iron with you.*

Early signs of iron overdose may not appear for up to 60 minutes or more. Do not delay going to the emergency room while waiting for signs to appear.

Side Effects of This Dietary Supplement

Along with its needed effects, a dietary supplement may cause some unwanted effects. Although not all of these effects may occur, if they do occur they may need medical attention.

Check with your health care professional if any of the following side effects occur:

More common—with the injection only

Backache or muscle pain; chest pain; chills; dizziness; fainting; fast heartbeat; fever with increased sweating; flushing; headache; metallic taste; nausea or vomiting; numbness, pain, or tingling of hands or feet; pain or redness at injection site; redness of skin; skin rash or hives; troubled breathing

More common—when taken by mouth only

Abdominal or stomach pain, cramping, or soreness (continuing)

Less common or rare—when taken by mouth only

Chest or throat pain, especially when swallowing; stools with signs of blood (red or black color)

Early symptoms of iron overdose

Diarrhea (may contain blood); nausea; stom-

ach pain or cramping (sharp); vomiting,
severe (may contain blood)

Note: Symptoms of iron overdose may not occur
for up to 60 minutes or more after the overdose was taken. By this time you should
have had emergency room treatment. Do
not delay going to emergency room while
waiting for signs to appear.

Late symptoms of iron overdose

Bluish-colored lips, fingernails, and palms of
hands; convulsions (seizures); drowsiness;
pale, clammy skin; unusual tiredness or
weakness; weak and fast heartbeat

Other side effects may occur that usually do
not need medical attention. These side effects
may go away during treatment as your body
adjusts to the dietary supplement. However,
check with your health care professional if
any of the following side effects continue or
are bothersome:

More common

Constipation; diarrhea; nausea; vomiting

Less common

Darkened urine; heartburn

Stools commonly become dark green or black
when iron preparations are taken by mouth.
This is caused by unabsorbed iron and is
harmless. However, in rare cases, black stools
of a sticky consistency may occur along with
other side effects such as red streaks in the
stool, cramping, soreness, or sharp pains in
the stomach or abdominal area. Check with
your health care professional immediately if
these side effects appear.

If you have been receiving injections of iron, you may notice a brown discoloration of your skin. This color usually fades within several weeks or months.

Other side effects not listed above may also occur in some individuals. If you notice any other effects, check with your health care professional.

MAGNESIUM
SUPPLEMENTS Systemic

Some commonly used brand names are:

In the U.S.—

Almora[4]
Chloromag[1]
Citroma[2]
Concentrated Phillips' Milk of Magnesia[5]
Mag-200[7]
Mag-L-100[1]
Magonate[4]
Mag-Ox 400[7]
Mag-Tab SR[6]

Magtrate[4]
Maox[7]
MGP[4]
Phillips' Chewable Tablets[5]
Phillips' Milk of Magnesia[5]
Slow-Mag[1]
Uro-Mag[7]

In Canada—

Citro-Mag[2]
Mag 2[8]
Maglucate[4]
Magnesium-Rougier[3]

Phillips' Magnesia Tablets[5]
Phillips' Milk of Magnesia[5]

Other commonly used names are:

Magnesium glucoheptonate[3]
Magnesium pyroglutamate[8]

Note: For quick reference, the following magnesium supplements are numbered to match the corresponding brand names.

This information applies to the following:

1. Magnesium Chloride (mag-NEE-zhum KLOR-ide)‡
2. Magnesium Citrate (SIH-trayt)‡
3. Magnesium Gluceptate (gloo-SEP-tate)*
4. Magnesium Gluconate (GLOO-ko-nate)‡
5. Magnesium Hydroxide (hye-DROX-ide)‡§
6. Magnesium Lactate (LAK-tate)†‡
7. Magnesium Oxide (OX-ide)‡
8. Magnesium Pidolate (PID-o-late)*
9. Magnesium Sulfate (SUL-fate)‡§

*Not commercially available in the U.S.
†Not commercially available in Canada.

‡Generic name product may be available in the U.S.
§Generic name product may be available in Canada.

Description

Magnesium is used as a dietary supplement for individuals who are deficient in magnesium. Although a balanced diet usually supplies all the magnesium a person needs, magnesium supplements may be needed by patients who have lost magnesium because of illness or treatment with certain medicines.

Lack of magnesium may lead to irritability, muscle weakness, and irregular heartbeat.

Injectable magnesium is administered only by or under the supervision of your health care professional. Some oral magnesium preparations are available only with a prescription. Other forms of magnesium are available without a prescription.

Magnesium supplements are available in the following dosage forms:

Oral

Magnesium Chloride
- Enteric-coated tablets (U.S.)
- Extended-release tablets (U.S.)

Magnesium Citrate
- Oral solution (U.S. and Canada)

Magnesium Gluceptate
- Oral solution (Canada)

Magnesium Gluconate
- Oral solution (U.S.)
- Tablets (U.S. and Canada)

Magnesium Hydroxide
- Tablets (U.S.)
- Chewable tablets (U.S. and Canada)
- Oral solution (U.S. and Canada)

Magnesium Lactate
- Extended-release tablets (U.S.)

Magnesium Oxide
- Capsules (U.S.)
- Tablets (U.S. and Canada)

Magnesium Pidolate
- Powder for oral solution (Canada)

Magnesium Sulfate
- Crystals (U.S.)

Parenteral

Magnesium Chloride
- Injection (U.S.)

Magnesium Sulfate
- Injection (U.S. and Canada)

Importance of Diet

The best dietary sources of magnesium include green leafy vegetables, nuts, peas, beans, and cereal grains in which the germ or outer layers have not been removed. Hard water has been found to contain more magnesium than soft water. A diet high in fat may cause less magnesium to be absorbed. Cooking may decrease the magnesium content of food.

Normal daily recommended intakes in milligrams (mg) for magnesium are generally defined as follows:

Persons	U.S. (mg)	Canada (mg)
Infants and children		
Birth to 3 years of age	40–80	20–50
4 to 6 years of age	120	65
7 to 10 years of age	170	100–135
Adolescent and adult males	270–400	130–250
Adolescent and adult females	280–300	135–210
Pregnant females	320	195–245
Breast-feeding females	340–355	245–265

Before Using This Dietary Supplement

If you are taking this dietary supplement without a prescription, carefully read and follow any precautions on the label. For magnesium supplements, the following should be considered:

Older adults—Studies have shown that older adults may have lower blood levels of magnesium than younger adults. Your health care professional may recommend that you take a magnesium supplement.

Medicines or other dietary supplements—Although certain medicines or other dietary supplements should not be used together at all, in other cases they may be used together even if an interaction might occur. In these cases, your health care professional may want to change the dose, or other precautions may be necessary. When you are taking magnesium, it is especially important that your health care professional know if you are taking any of the following:

- Cellulose sodium phosphate—Use with magnesium supplements may prevent cellulose sodium phosphate from working properly; magnesium supplements should be taken at least 1 hour before or after cellulose sodium phosphate

- Magnesium-containing preparations, other, including magnesium enemas—Use with magnesium supplements may cause high blood levels of magnesium, which may increase the chance of side effects

- Sodium polystyrene sulfonate—Use with magnesium supplements may cause the magnesium supplement to be less effective

- Tetracyclines, oral—Use with magnesium supplements may prevent the tetracycline from working properly; magnesium supplements should be taken at least 1 to 3 hours before or after oral tetracycline

Other medical problems—The presence of other medical problems may affect the use of magnesium. Make sure you tell your health care professional if you have any other medical problems, especially:

- Heart disease—Magnesium supplements may make this condition worse

- Kidney problems—Magnesium supplements may increase the risk of hypermagnesemia (too much magnesium in the blood), which could cause serious side effects; your health care professional may need to change your dose

Proper Use of This Dietary Supplement
Magnesium supplements should be taken with meals. Taking magnesium supplements on an empty stomach may cause diarrhea.

For individuals taking the *extended-release form* of this dietary supplement:

- Swallow the tablets whole. Do not chew or suck on the tablet.
- Some tablets may be broken or crushed and sprinkled on applesauce or other soft food. However, check with your health care professional first, since this should not be done for most tablets.

For individuals taking the *powder form* of this dietary supplement:

- Pour powder into a glass.
- Add water and stir.

Side Effects of This Dietary Supplement
Along with its needed effects, a dietary supplement may cause some unwanted effects. Although not all of these side effects may occur, if they do occur they may need medical attention.

Check with your health care professional immediately if any of the following side effects occur:
   Rare (with injectable magnesium only)
      Dizziness or fainting; flushing; irritation and
         pain at injection site—for intramuscular

administration only; muscle paralysis; troubled breathing

Symptoms of overdose (rare in individuals with normal kidney function)

Blurred or double vision; coma; dizziness or fainting; drowsiness (severe); increased or decreased urination; slow heartbeat; troubled breathing

Other side effects may occur that usually do not need medical attention. These side effects may go away during treatment as your body adjusts to the dietary supplement. However, check with your health care professional if the following side effect continues or is bothersome:

Less common (with oral magnesium)

Diarrhea

Other side effects not listed above may also occur in some individuals. If you notice any other effects, check with your health care professional.

MANGANESE SUPPLEMENTS Systemic

This information applies to the following:

1. Manganese Chloride (MAN-ga-nees KLOR-ide)†‡
2. Manganese Sulfate (SUL-fate)†

†Not commercially available in Canada.

‡Generic name product may also be available in the U.S.

Description

Manganese supplements are used to prevent or treat manganese deficiency.

The body needs manganese for normal growth and health. For patients who are unable to get enough manganese in their regular diet or who have a need for more manganese, manganese supplements may be necessary. Manganese helps your body metabolize fat, carbohydrates, and proteins. It does so as part of several enzymes.

Manganese deficiency has not been reported in humans. Lack of manganese in animals has been found to cause improper formation of bone and cartilage, may decrease the body's ability to use sugar properly, and may cause growth problems.

Injectable manganese supplements are given by or under the supervision of a health care professional.

Manganese supplements are available in the following dosage forms:

Oral

    Manganese is available orally as part of a multivitamin/mineral combination.

Parenteral

Manganese Chloride
- Injection (U.S.)

Manganese Sulfate
- Injection (U.S.)

Importance of Diet

Manganese is found in whole grains, cereal products, lettuce, dry beans, and peas.

Normal daily recommended intakes for manganese are generally defined as follows:

- Infants and children—
  Birth to 3 years of age: 0.3 to 1.5 milligrams (mg).
  4 to 6 years of age: 1.5 to 2 mg.
  7 to 10 years of age: 2 to 3 mg.
- Adolescents and adults—2 to 5 mg.

Before Using This Dietary Supplement

If you are taking this dietary supplement without a prescription, carefully read and follow any precautions on the label. For manganese, the following should be considered:

Other medical problems—The presence of other medical problems may affect the use of

manganese. Make sure you tell your doctor if you have any other medical problems, especially:

- Biliary disease or
- Liver disease—Taking manganese supplements may cause high blood levels of manganese, and dosage of manganese may have to be changed

---

Side Effects of This Dietary Supplement

No side effects or toxic effects have been reported for manganese. However, check with your health care professional if you notice any unusual effects while you are taking it.

MOLYBDENUM SUPPLEMENTS Systemic[†]

A commonly used brand name in the U.S. is Molypen. Generic name product may also be available.

---

†Not commercially available in Canada.

Description

The body needs molybdenum (moh-LIB-denum) for normal growth and health. For patients who are unable to get enough molybdenum in their regular diet or who have a need for more molybdenum, molybdenum supplements may be necessary. They are generally taken by mouth in multivitamin/mineral products, but some patients may have to receive them by injection. Molybdenum is part of certain enzymes that are important for several body functions.

A deficiency of molybdenum is rare. However, if the body does not get enough molybdenum, certain enzymes needed by the body are affected. This may lead to a buildup of unwanted substances in some people.

Injectable molybdenum is administered only by or under the supervision of your health care professional. Molybdenum is available in the following dosage forms:

Oral

Molybdenum is available orally as part of a multivitamin/mineral combination.

Parenteral
* Injection (U.S.)

Importance of Diet

The amount of molybdenum in foods depends on the soil in which the food is grown. Some soils have more molybdenum than others. Peas, beans, cereal products, leafy vegetables, and low-fat milk are good sources of molybdenum.

Normal daily recommended intakes for molybdenum are generally defined as follows:

* Infants and children—
  Birth to 3 years of age: 15 to 50 micrograms (mcg).
  4 to 6 years of age: 30 to 75 mcg.
  7 to 10 years of age: 50 to 150 mcg.
* Adolescents and adults—75 to 250 mcg.

Before Using This Dietary Supplement

If you are taking this dietary supplement without a prescription, carefully read and follow any precautions on the label. For molybdenum, the following should be considered:

Other medical problems—The presence of other medical problems may affect the use of molybdenum. Make sure you tell your health care professional if you have any other medical problems, especially:

- Copper deficiency—Molybdenum may make this condition worse
- Kidney disease or
- Liver disease—These conditions may cause higher blood levels of molybdenum, which may increase the chance of unwanted effects

---

Side Effects of This Dietary Supplement

Along with its needed effects, a dietary supplement may cause some unwanted effects. Although oral molybdenum supplements have not been reported to cause any side effects, *check with your health care professional immediately* if any of the following side effects occur:

Symptoms of overdose

Joint pain; side, lower back, or stomach pain; swelling of feet or lower legs

Note: Reported rarely in individuals consuming foods grown in soil containing a high content of molybdenum.

Other side effects not listed above may also occur in some individuals. If you notice any other effects, check with your health care professional.

NIACIN (Vitamin B₃)   Systemic

Some commonly used brand names are:

In the U.S.

Endur-Acin[1]	Nico-400[1]
Nia-Bid[1]	Nicobid Tempules[1]
Niac[1]	Nicolar[1]
Niacels[1]	Nicotinex Elixir[1]
Niacor[1]	Slo-Niacin[1]

Generic name product may also be available.

In Canada

Novo-Niacin[1]

Generic name product may also be available.

Other commonly used names are:

Nicotinamide[2]	Vitamin B₃[1,2]
Nicotinic acid[1]	

Note: For quick reference, the following products are numbered to match the corresponding brand names.

This information applies to the following products:

1. Niacin (nye-a-SIN)‡§
2. Niacinamide (nye-a-SIN-a-mide)‡§

---

‡Generic name product may also be available in the U.S.

§Generic name product may also be available in Canada.

Description

Vitamins (VYE-ta-mins) are compounds that you *must* have for growth and health. They are needed in small amounts only and are usually available in the foods that you eat. Niacin (NYE-a-sin) is necessary for many normal functions of the body, including normal tissue metabolism. It may have other effects as well.

Lack of niacin may lead to a condition called pellagra. Pellegra causes diarrhea, stomach problems, skin problems, sores in the mouth, anemia (weak blood), and mental problems. Your health care professional may treat this by prescribing niacin for you.

Some conditions may increase your need for niacin. These include:

- Cancer
- Diabetes mellitus (sugar diabetes)
- Diarrhea (prolonged)
- Fever (prolonged)
- Hartnup disease
- Infection (prolonged)
- Intestinal problems
- Liver disease
- Mouth or throat sores
- Overactive thyroid
- Pancreas disease
- Stomach ulcer
- Stress (prolonged)
- Surgical removal of stomach

Increased need for niacin should be determined by your health care professional.

Injectable niacin is administered only by or under the supervision of your health care professional. Other forms of niacin are available without a prescription.

Niacin and niacinamide are available in the following dosage forms:

Oral

Niacin
- Extended-release capsules (U.S.)
- Solution (U.S.)
- Tablets (U.S. and Canada)
- Extended-release tablets (U.S. and Canada)

Niacinamide
- Tablets (U.S. and Canada)

Parenteral

Niacin
- Injection (U.S.)

Niacinamide
- Injection (U.S.)

Importance of Diet

Niacin is found in meats, eggs, and milk and dairy products. Little niacin is lost from foods during ordinary cooking.

Normal daily recommended intakes in milligrams (mg) for niacin are generally defined as follows:

Persons	U.S. (mg)	Canada (mg)
Infants and children		
Birth to 3 years of age	5–9	4–9
4 to 6 years of age	12	13
7 to 10 years of age	13	14–18
Adolescent and adult males	15–20	14–23
Adolescent and adult females	13–15	14–16
Pregnant females	17	14–16
Breast-feeding females	20	14–16

Before Using This Dietary Supplement
If you are taking this dietary supplement without a prescription, carefully read and follow any precautions on the label. For niacin or niacinamide, the following should be considered:

Other medical problems—The presence of other medical problems may affect the use of niacin or niacinamide. Make sure you tell your health care professional if you have any other medical problems, especially:

- Bleeding problems or
- Diabetes mellitus (sugar diabetes) or
- Glaucoma or
- Gout or
- Liver disease or
- Low blood pressure or
- Stomach ulcer—Niacin or niacinamide may make these conditions worse

---

Proper Use of This Dietary Supplement
If this dietary supplement upsets your stomach, it may be taken with meals or milk. If stomach upset (nausea or diarrhea) continues, check with your health care professional.

For individuals taking the *extended-release capsule form* of this dietary supplement:

- Swallow the capsule whole. Do not crush, break, or chew before swallowing. However, if the capsule is too large to swallow, you may mix the contents of the capsule with jam or jelly and swallow without chewing.

For individuals taking the *extended-release tablet form* of this dietary supplement:

*   Swallow the tablet whole. If the tablet is scored, it may be broken, but not crushed or chewed, before being swallowed.

Side Effects of This Dietary Supplement

Along with its needed effects, a dietary supplement may cause some unwanted effects. Although not all of these side effects may occur, if they do occur they may need medical attention.

Check with your health care professional immediately if any of the following side effects occur:

With injection only

Skin rash or itching; wheezing

With prolonged use of extended-release niacin

Darkening of urine; light gray-colored stools; loss of appetite; severe stomach pain; yellow eyes or skin

Other side effects may occur that usually do not need medical attention. These side effects may go away during treatment as your body adjusts to the dietary supplement. However, check with your health care professional if any of the following side effects continue or are bothersome:

Less common—with niacin only

Feeling of warmth; flushing or redness of
skin, especially on face and neck; headache

With high doses

Diarrhea; dizziness or faintness; dryness of
skin; fever; frequent urination; itching of
skin; joint pain; muscle aching or cramping; nausea or vomiting; side, lower back,
or stomach pain; swelling of feet or lower
legs; unusual thirst; unusual tiredness or
weakness; unusually fast, slow, or irregular heartbeat

Other side effects not listed above may also
occur in some individuals. If you notice any
other effects, check with your health care
professional.

Other Claimed Uses

Claims that niacin is effective for treatment
of acne, alcoholism, unwanted effects of drug
abuse, leprosy, motion sickness, muscle problems, poor circulation, and mental problems,
and for prevention of heart attacks, have not
been proven. Many of these treatments involve large and expensive amounts of
vitamins.

PANTOTHENIC ACID
(Vitamin B₅)   Systemic†

Other commonly used names are vitamin B_5 and calcium pantothenate.

Generic name product may also be available in the U.S.

---

†Not commercially available in Canada.

Description

Vitamins (VYE-ta-mins) are compounds that you *must* have for growth and health. They are needed in only small amounts and are usually available in the foods that you eat. Pantothenic acid (pan-toh-THEN-ik AS-id) (vitamin B_5) is needed for metabolism of carbohydrates, proteins, and fats.

No problems have been found that are due to a lack of pantothenic acid alone. However, a lack of one B vitamin usually goes along with a lack of others, so pantothenic acid is often included in B complex products.

Pantothenic acid is available without a prescription in the following dosage forms:

Oral

Calcium pantothenate
- Tablets (U.S.)

Pantothenic acid
- Capsules (U.S.)
- Oral solution (U.S.)
- Tablets (U.S.)
- Extended-release tablets (U.S.)

Importance of Diet

Pantothenic acid is found in various foods including peas and beans (except green beans), lean meat, poultry, fish, and whole-grain cereals. Little pantothenic acid is lost from foods with ordinary cooking.

Normal daily recommended intakes for pantothenic acid are generally defined as follows:

- Infants and children—
  Birth to 3 years of age: 2 to 3 milligrams (mg).
  4 to 6 years of age: 3 to 4 mg.
  7 to 10 years of age: 4 to 5 mg.
- Adolescents and adults—4 to 7 mg.

Side Effects of This Dietary Supplement

Along with its needed effects, a dietary supplement may cause some unwanted effects. Although pantothenic acid does not usually cause any side effects, check with your health care professional if you notice any unusual effects while you are taking it.

Other Claimed Uses

Claims that pantothenic acid is effective for treatment of nerve damage, breathing problems, itching and other skin problems, and poisoning with some other drugs; for getting rid of or preventing gray hair; for preventing arthritis, allergies, and birth defects; or for improving mental ability have not been proven.

PHOSPHATES Systemic

Some commonly used brand names are:

In the U.S.—

K-Phos M. F.[2] Neutra-Phos[2]

K-Phos Neutral[2] Neutra-Phos-K[1]

K-Phos No. 2[2] Uro-KP-Neutral[2]

K-Phos Original[1]

In Canada—

Uro-KP-Neutral[2]

Note: For quick reference, the following phosphates are numbered to match the corresponding brand names.

This information applies to the following:

1. Potassium Phosphates (poe-TASS-ee-um FOS-fates)‡§
2. Potassium and Sodium (SOE-dee-um) Phosphates
3. Sodium Phosphates†‡

---

†Not commercially available in Canada.

‡Generic name product may also be available in the U.S.

§Generic name product may also be available in Canada.

Description

Phosphates are used as dietary supplements for patients who are unable to get enough phosphorus in their regular diet, usually because of certain illnesses or diseases. Phosphate is the drug form (salt) of phosphorus. Some phosphates are used to make the urine more acid, which helps treat certain urinary tract infections.

Injectable phosphates are administered only by or under the supervision of your health care professional. Some of these oral preparations are available only with a prescription. Others are available without a prescription. You should take phosphates only under the supervision of your health care professional.

Phosphates are available in the following dosage forms:

Oral

Potassium Phosphates
- Capsules for solution (U.S.)
- Powder for solution (U.S.)
- Tablets for solution (U.S.)

Potassium and Sodium Phosphates
- Capsules for solution (U.S.)
- Powder for solution (U.S.)
- Tablets for solution (U.S. and Canada)

Parenteral

Potassium Phosphates
- Injection (U.S. and Canada)

Sodium Phosphates
- Injection (U.S.)

Importance of Diet

The best dietary sources of phosphorus include dairy products, meat, poultry, fish, and cereal products.

Normal daily recommended intakes in milligrams (mg) for phosphorus are generally defined as follows:

Persons	U.S. (mg)	Canada (mg)
Infants and children		
Birth to 3 years of age	300–800	150–350
4 to 6 years of age	800	400
7 to 10 years of age	800	500–800
Adolescent and adult males	800–1200	700–1000
Adolescent and adult females	800–1200	800–850
Pregnant females	1200	1050
Breast-feeding females	1200	1050

Before Using Phosphates

In deciding to use phosphates, the risks of taking them must be weighed against the good they will do. This is a decision you and your health care professional will make. For phosphates the following should be considered:

Children—Use of enemas that contain phosphates in children has resulted in high blood levels of phosphorus.

Medicines or other dietary supplements—Although certain medicines or dietary supplements should not be used together at all, in other cases they may be used together even if an interaction might occur. In these cases, your health care professional may want to change the dose, or other precautions may be necessary. When you are taking phosphates, it is especially important that your health care professional know if you are taking any of the following:

- Amiloride (e.g., Midamor) or
- Angiotensin-converting enzyme (ACE) inhibitors (benazepril [e.g., Lotensin], captopril [e.g., Capoten], enalapril [e.g., Vasotec], fosinopril [e.g., Monopril], lisinopril [e.g., Zestril, Prinivil], quinapril [e.g., Accupril], ramipril [e.g., Altace]) or
- Cyclosporine
- Digitalis glycosides (heart medicine) or
- Heparin (e.g., Panheprin), with long-term use, or
- Medicine for inflammation or pain (except narcotics) or
- Other potassium-containing medicine or
- Salt substitutes, low-salt foods, or milk or
- Spironolactone (e.g., Aldactone) or
- Triamterene (e.g., Dyrenium)—Use with potassium-containing phosphates may increase the risk of hyperkalemia (too much potassium in the blood), possibly leading to serious side effects
- Antacids—Use with phosphates may prevent the phosphate from working properly
- Calcium-containing medicine, including antacids and calcium supplements—Use with phosphates may prevent the phosphate from working properly; calcium deposits may form in tissues
- Corticosteroids (cortisone-like medicine)—Use with sodium-containing phosphates may increase the risk of swelling
- Phosphate-containing medications, other, including phosphate enemas—Use with sodium or potassium phophates may cause

high blood levels of phosphorus, which may increase the chance of side effects

- Sodium-containing medicines (other)—Use with sodium phosphates may cause your body to retain (keep) water

Other medical problems—The presence of other medical problems may affect the use of phosphates. Make sure you tell your health care professional if you have any other medical problems, especially:

- Burns, severe or
- Heart disease or
- Pancreatitis (inflammation of the pancreas) or
- Rickets or
- Softening of bones or
- Underactive parathyroid glands—Sodium- or potassium-containing phosphates may make these conditions worse
- Dehydration or
- Underactive adrenal glands—Potassium-containing phosphates may increase the risk of hyperkalemia (too much potassium in the blood)
- Edema (swelling in feet or lower legs or fluid in lungs) or
- High blood pressure or
- Liver disease or
- Toxemia of pregnancy—Sodium-containing phosphates may make these conditions worse
- High blood levels of phosphate (hyperphosphatemia)—Use of phosphates may make this condition worse
- Infected kidney stones—Phosphates may make this condition worse
- Kidney disease—Sodium-containing phos-

phates may make this condition worse; potassium-containing phosphates may increase the risk of hyperkalemia (too much potassium in the blood)

- Myotonia congenita—Potassium-containing phosphates may increase the risk of hyperkalemia (too much potassium in the blood), and make this condition worse

---

Proper Use of Phosphates

For patients taking the *tablet form* of phosphates:

- *Do not swallow the tablet.* Before taking, dissolve the tablet in ¾ to 1 glass (6 to 8 ounces) of water. Let the tablet soak in water for 2 to 5 minutes and then stir until completely dissolved.

For patients using the *capsule form* of phosphates:

- *Do not swallow the capsule.* Before taking, mix the contents of 1 capsule in one-third glass (about 2½ ounces) of water or juice or the contents of 2 capsules in two-thirds glass (about 5 ounces) of water and stir well until dissolved.

For patients using the *powder form* of phosphates:

- Add the entire contents of 1 bottle (2¼ ounces) to enough warm water to make 1 gallon of solution *or* the contents of one packet to enough warm water to make 1/3 of a glass (about 2.5 ounces) of solution. Shake the container for 2 or 3 minutes or until all the powder is dissolved.

- Do not dilute solution further.
- This solution may be chilled to improve the flavor; do not allow it to freeze.
- Discard unused solution after 60 days.

Take phosphates immediately after meals or with food to lessen possible stomach upset or laxative action.

Precautions While Using Phosphates

Do not take iron supplements within 1 to 2 hours of taking this medicine. To do so may keep the iron from working properly.

For patients taking potassium phosphate:

- Check with your health care professional before starting any strenuous physical exercise, especially if you are out of condition and are taking other medication. Exercise and certain medicines may increase the amount of potassium in the blood.

For patients on a *potassium-restricted diet:*

- Potassium phosphates may contain a large amount of potassium. If you have any questions about this, check with your health care professional.

- Do not use salt substitutes and low-salt milk unless told to do so by your health

care professional. They may contain
potassium.

For patients on a sodium-restricted diet:
- Sodium phosphates may contain a large
  amount of sodium. If you have any questions about this, check with your health
  care professional.

Side Effects of Phosphates

Along with its needed effects, phosphates
may cause some unwanted effects. Although
not all of these side effects may occur, if they
do occur they may need medical attention.

Check with your health care professional as
soon as possible if any of the following side
effects occur:

Less common or rare

Confusion; convulsions (seizures); decrease
in amount of urine or in frequency of urination; fast, slow, or irregular heartbeat;
headache or dizziness; increased thirst;
muscle cramps; numbness, tingling, pain,
or weakness in hands or feet; numbness or
tingling around lips; shortness of breath
or troubled breathing; swelling of feet or
lower legs; tremor; unexplained anxiety;
unusual tiredness or weakness; weakness
or heaviness of legs; weight gain

Other side effects may occur that usually do
not need medical attention. These side effects
may go away during treatment as your body
adjusts to the phosphates. However, check

with your health care professional if any of the following side effects continue or are bothersome:

Diarrhea; nausea or vomiting; stomach pain

Other side effects not listed above may also occur in some patients. If you notice any other effects, check with your health care professional.

POTASSIUM SUPPLEMENTS Systemic

Some commonly used brand names are:

In the U.S.—

Cena-K[5]
Effer-K[4]
Gen-K[5]
Glu-K[6]
K-8[5]
K+ 10[5]
Kaochlor 10%[5]
Kaochlor S-F 10%[5]
Kaon[7]
Kaon-Cl[5]
Kaon-Cl-10[5]
Kaon-Cl 20% Liquid[5]
Kato[5]
Kay Ciel[5]
Kaylixir[6]
K+ Care[5]
K+ Care ET[2]
K-Dur[5]
K-Electrolyte[2]
K-G Elixir[6]
K-Ide[2,5]
K-Lease[5]
K-Lor[5]
Klor-Con 8[5]
Klor-Con 10[5]
Klor-Con/EF[2]

Klor-Con Powder[5]
Klor-Con/25 Powder[5]
Klorvess[3]
Klorvess Effervescent Granules[3]
Klorvess 10% Liquid[5]
Klotrix[5]
K-Lyte[2]
K-Lyte/Cl[3]
K-Lyte/Cl 50[3]
K-Lyte/Cl Powder[5]
K-Lyte DS[4]
K-Norm[5]
Kolyum[7]
K-Sol[5]
K-Tab[5]
K-Vescent[2]
Micro-K[5]
Micro-K 10[5]
Micro-K LS[5]
Potasalan[5]
Rum-K[5]
Slow-K[5]
Ten-K[5]
Tri-K[9]
Twin-K[8]

In Canada—

Apo-K[5]
K-10[5]
Kalium Durules[5]
Kaochlor-10[5]
Kaochlor-20[5]
Kaon[6]
KCL 5%[5]
K-Dur[5]

K-Long[5]
K-Lor[5]
K-Lyte[2]
K-Lyte/Cl[5]
K-Med 900[5]
Micro-K[5]
Micro-K 10[5]
Neo-K[3]

In Canada (cont'd)—

Potassium-Rougier[6]   Roychlor-10%[5]
Potassium-Sandoz[3]   Slow-K[5]

Another commonly used name for trikates is potassium triplex.

Note: For quick reference, the following potassium supplements are numbered to match the corresponding brand names.

This information applies to the following:

1. Potassium Acetate (poe-TAS-ee-um AS-a-tate)‡†
2. Potassium Bicarbonate (bi-KAR-bo-nate)‡
3. Potassium Bicarbonate and Potassium Chloride (KLOR-ide)
4. Potassium Bicarbonate and Potassium Citrate (SIH-trayt)†
5. Potassium Chloride‡§
6. Potassium Gluconate (GLOO-ko-nate)‡
7. Potassium Gluconate and Potassium Chloride†
8. Potassium Gluconate and Potassium Citrate†
9. Trikates (TRI-kates)†

---

†Not commercially available in Canada.
‡Generic name product may be available in the U.S.
§Generic name product may be available in Canada.

Description

Potassium is needed to maintain good health. Although a balanced diet usually supplies all the potassium a person needs, potassium supplements may be needed by patients who do not have enough potassium in their regular diet or have lost too much potassium because of illness or treatment with certain medicines.

Lack of potassium may cause muscle weakness, irregular heartbeat, mood changes, or nausea and vomiting.

Injectable potassium is administered only by or under the supervision of your doctor. Some forms of oral potassium may be available in stores without a prescription. Since too much potassium may cause health problems, you should take potassium supplements only if directed by your doctor. Potassium supplements are available with your doctor's prescription in the following dosage forms:

Oral

Potassium Bicarbonate
   • Tablets for solution (U.S. and Canada)
Potassium Bicarbonate and Potassium Chloride
   • Powder for solution (U.S. and Canada)
   • Tablets for solution (U.S. and Canada)
Potassium Bicarbonate and Potassium Citrate
   • Tablets for solution (U.S.)
Potassium Chloride
   • Extended-release capsules (U.S. and Canada)
   • Solution (U.S. and Canada)
   • Powder for solution (U.S. and Canada)
   • Powder for suspension (U.S.)
   • Extended-release tablets (U.S. and Canada)
Potassium Gluconate
   • Elixir (U.S. and Canada)
   • Tablets (U.S.)
Potassium Gluconate and Potassium Chloride
   • Solution (U.S.)
   • Powder for solution (U.S.)
Potassium Gluconate and Potassium Citrate
   • Solution (U.S.)
Trikates
   • Solution (U.S.)

Parenteral

Potassium Acetate
   • Injection (U.S.)

Potassium Chloride
   • Concentrate for injection (U.S. and
     Canada)

Importance of Diet

The following table includes some potassium-rich foods:

Food (amount)	Milligrams of potassium	Milli-equivalents of potassium
Acorn squash, cooked (1 cup)	896	23
Potato with skin, baked (1 long)	844	22
Spinach, cooked (1 cup)	838	21
Lentils, cooked (1 cup)	731	19
Kidney beans, cooked (1 cup)	713	18
Split peas, cooked (1 cup)	710	18
White navy beans, cooked (1 cup)	669	17
Butternut squash, cooked (1 cup)	583	15
Watermelon (1/16)	560	14
Raisins (1/2 cup)	553	14
Yogurt, low-fat, plain (1 cup)	531	14
Orange juice, frozen (1 cup)	503	13
Brussel sprouts, cooked (1 cup)	494	13
Zucchini, cooked, sliced (1 cup)	456	12
Banana (medium)	451	12
Collards, frozen, cooked (1 cup)	427	11
Cantaloupe (1/4)	412	11
Milk, low-fat 1% (1 cup)	348	9
Broccoli, frozen, cooked (1 cup)	332	9

Lack of potassium is rare. It is thought that 1600 to 2000 milligrams (mg) (40 to 50 milliequivalents [mEq]) of potassium a day for adults is adequate.

Remember:
- The total amount of potassium that you get every day includes what you get from food *and* what you may take as a supplement. Read the labels of processed foods. Many foods now have added potassium.
- Your total intake of potassium should not be greater than the recommended amounts, unless ordered by your health care professional. In some cases, too much potassium may cause muscle weakness, confusion, irregular heartbeat, or difficult breathing.

Before Using This Potassium Supplement

In deciding to use a potassium supplement, the risks of taking it must be weighed against the good it will do. This is a decision you and your health care professional will make. For potassium supplements, the following should be considered:

Older adults—Older adults may be at a greater risk of developing high blood levels of potassium (hyperkalemia). Follow your health care professional's orders carefully when you are taking potassium supplements.

Other medicines—Although certain medicines and potassium supplements should not be used together at all, in other cases they may be used together even if an interaction might occur. In these cases, your health care professional may want to change the dose, or other precautions may be necessary. When you are taking potassium supplements, it is especially important that your health care professional know if you are taking any of the following:

* Amantadine (e.g., Symmetrel) or
* Anticholinergics (medicine for abdominal or stomach spasms or cramps) or
* Antidepressants (medicine for depression) or
* Antidyskinetics (medicine for Parkinson's disease or other conditions affecting control of muscles) or
* Antihistamines or
* Antipsychotic medicine (medicine for mental illness) or
* Buclizine (e.g., Bucladin) or
* Carbamazepine (e.g., Tegretol) or
* Cyclizine (e.g., Marezine) or
* Cyclobenzaprine (e.g., Flexeril) or
* Disopyramide (e.g., Norpace) or
* Flavoxate (e.g., Urispas) or
* Ipratropium (e.g., Atrovent) or
* Meclizine (e.g., Antivert) or
* Methylphenidate (e.g., Ritalin) or
* Orphenadrine (e.g., Norflex) or
* Oxybutynin (e.g., Ditropan) or
* Procainamide (e.g., Pronestyl) or
* Promethazine (e.g., Phenergan) or
* Quinidine (e.g., Quinidex) or
* Trimeprazine (e.g., Temaril)—Use with po-

tassium supplements may cause or worsen certain stomach or intestine problems

- Angiotensin-converting enzyme (ACE) inhibitors (benazepril [e.g., Lotensin], captopril [e.g., Capoten], enalapril [e.g., Vasotec], fosinopril [e.g., Monotril], lisinopril [e.g., Prinivil, Zestril], quinapril [e.g., Accupril], ramipril [e.g., Altace]) or
- Amiloride (e.g., Midamor) or
- Beta-adrenergic blocking agents (acebutolol [e.g., Sectral], atenolol [e.g., Tenormin], betaxolol [e.g., Kerlone], carteolol [e.g., Cartrol], labetalol [e.g., Normodyne], metoprolol [e.g., Lopressor], nadolol [e.g., Corgard], oxprenolol [e.g., Trasicor], penbutolol [e.g., Levatol], pindolol [e.g., Visken], propranolol [e.g., Inderal], sotalol [e.g., Sotacor], timolol [e.g., Blocadren]) or
- Heparin (e.g., Panheprin) or
- Inflammation or pain medicine (except narcotics) or
- Potassium-containing medicines (other) or
- Salt substitutes, low-salt foods, or milk or
- Spironolactone (e.g., Aldactone) or
- Triamterene (e.g., Dyrenium)—Use with potassium supplements may further increase potassium blood levels, which may cause or worsen heart problems
- Digitalis glycosides (heart medicine)—Use with potassium supplements may make heart problems worse
- Thiazide diuretics (water pills)—If you have been taking a potassium supplement and a thiazide diuretic together, stopping the thiazide diuretic may cause hyperkalemia (high blood levels of potassium)

Other medical problems—The presence of other medical problems may affect the use of

potassium supplements. Make sure you tell
your health care professional if you have any
other medical problems, especially:

- Addison's disease (underactive adrenal
  glands) or
- Dehydration (excessive loss of body water,
  continuing or severe) or
- Diabetes mellitus or
- Kidney disease—Potassium supplements may
  increase the risk of hyperkalemia (high blood
  levels of potassium), which may worsen or
  cause heart problems in patients with these
  conditions
- Diarrhea (continuing or severe)—The loss of
  fluid in combination with potassium supplements may cause kidney problems, which
  may increase the risk of hyperkalemia (high
  blood levels of potassium)
- Heart disease—Potassium supplements may
  make this condition worse
- Intestinal or esophageal blockage—Potassium
  supplements may damage the intestines
- Stomach ulcer—Potassium supplements may
  make this condition worse

Proper Use of This
Potassium Supplement

For patients taking the *liquid form* of this potassium supplement:

- This potassium supplement *must be di-
  luted* in at least one-half glass (4 ounces)
  of cold water or juice to reduce its possible stomach-irritating or laxative effect.
- If you are on a salt (sodium)-restricted

diet, check with your health care professional before using tomato juice to dilute your potassium supplement. Tomato juice has a high salt content.

For patients taking the *soluble granule, soluble powder, or soluble tablet form* of this potassium supplement:

- This potassium supplement *must be completely dissolved* in at least one-half glass (4 ounces) of cold water or juice to reduce its possible stomach-irritating or laxative effect.

- Allow any "fizzing" to stop before taking the dissolved potassium supplement.

- If you are on a salt (sodium)-restricted diet, check with your health care professional before using tomato juice to dilute your potassium supplement. Tomato juice has a high salt content.

For patients taking the *extended-release tablet form* of this potassium supplement:

- Swallow the tablets whole with a full (8-ounce) glass of water. Do not chew or suck on the tablet.

- Some tablets may be broken or crushed and sprinkled on applesauce or other soft food. However, check with your health care professional first, since this should not be done for most tablets.

- If you have trouble swallowing tablets or if they seem to stick in your throat, check with your health care professional. When potassium is not properly released, it can cause irritation that may lead to ulcers.

For patients taking the *extended-release capsule form* of this potassium supplement:

- Do not crush or chew the capsule. Swallow the capsule whole with a full (8-ounce) glass of water.
- Some capsules may be opened and the contents sprinkled on applesauce or other soft food. However, check with your health care professional first, since this should not be done for most capsules.

Take this potassium supplement immediately after meals or with food to lessen possible stomach upset or laxative action.

Take this potassium supplement only as directed by your health care professional. Do not take more of it, do not take it more often, and do not take it for a longer time than your health care professional ordered. *This is especially important if you are also taking both diuretics (water pills) and digitalis medicines for your heart.*

Missed dose—If you miss a dose of this potassium supplement and remember within 2 hours, take the missed dose right away with food or liquids. Then go back to your regular dosing schedule. However, if you do not remember until later, skip the missed dose and go back to your regular dosing schedule. Do not double doses.

Precautions While Using This Potassium Supplement

Your health care professional should check your progress at regular visits to make sure the potassium supplement is working properly and that possible side effects are avoided. Laboratory tests may be necessary.

Do not use salt substitutes, eat low-sodium foods, especially some breads and canned foods, or drink low-sodium milk unless you are told to do so by your health care professional, since these products may contain potassium. It is important to read the labels carefully on all low-sodium food products.

Check with your health care professional before starting any physical exercise program, especially if you are out of condition and are taking any other medicine. Exercise and certain medicines may increase the amount of potassium in the blood.

Check with your health care professional at once if you notice blackish stools or other signs of stomach or intestinal bleeding. This potassium supplement may cause such a condition to become worse, especially when taken in tablet form.

Side Effects of This Potassium Supplement

Along with its needed effects, a potassium supplement may cause some unwanted effects. Although not all of these side effects may occur, if they do occur they may need medical attention.

Stop taking this potassium supplement and check with your health care professional immediately if any of the following side effects occur:

Less common
> Confusion; irregular or slow heartbeat; numbness or tingling in hands, feet, or lips; shortness of breath or difficult breathing; unexplained anxiety; unusual tiredness or weakness; weakness or heaviness of legs

Also, check with your health care professional if any of the following side effects occur:

Rare
> Abdominal or stomach pain, cramping, or soreness (continuing); chest or throat pain, especially when swallowing; stools with signs of blood (red or black color)

Other side effects may occur that usually do not need medical attention. These side effects may go away during treatment as your body adjusts to the potassium supplement. However, check with your health care professional if any of the following side effects continue or are bothersome:

More common
> Diarrhea; nausea; stomach pain, discomfort, or gas (mild); vomiting

Sometimes you may see what appears to be a whole tablet in the stool after taking certain extended-release potassium chloride tablets.

This is to be expected. Your body has absorbed the potassium from the tablet and the shell is then expelled.

Other side effects not listed above may also occur in some patients. If you notice any other effects, check with your health care professional.

Other Claimed Uses

There is no evidence that potassium supplements are useful in the treatment of high blood pressure.

PYRIDOXINE
(Vitamin B₆) Systemic

Some commonly used brand names are:

In the U.S.—

Beesix	Pyri
Doxine	Rodex
Nestrex	Vitabee 6

Generic name product may also be available.

In Canada—

Generic name product is available.

Description

Vitamins (VYE-ta-mins) are compounds that you *must* have for growth and health. They are needed in small amounts only and are usually available in the foods that you eat. Pyridoxine (peer-i-DOX-een) (vitamin B₆) is necessary for normal metabolism of proteins, carbohydrates, and fats.

Some conditions may increase your need for pyridoxine. These include:

- Alcoholism
- Burns
- Diarrhea
- Dialysis
- Heart disease
- Intestinal problems
- Liver disease
- Overactive thyroid

- Stress, long-term illness, or serious injury
- Surgical removal of stomach

In addition, infants receiving unfortified formulas such as evaporated milk may need additional pyridoxine.

Increased need for pyridoxine should be determined by your health care professional.

Lack of pyridoxine may lead to anemia (weak blood), nerve damage, seizures, skin problems, and sores in the mouth. Your doctor may treat these problems by prescribing pyridoxine for you.

Injectable pyridoxine is administered only by or under the supervision of your health care professional. Oral forms of pyridoxine are available without a prescription.

Pyridoxine is available in the following dosage forms:

Oral

- Extended-release capsules (U.S.)
- Tablets (U.S. and Canada)
- Extended-release tablets (U.S.)

Parenteral

- Injection (U.S. and Canada)

Importance of Diet

Pyridoxine is found in various foods, including meats, bananas, lima beans, egg yolks, peanuts, and whole-grain cereals. Pyridoxine is not lost from food during ordinary cooking, although some other forms of vitamin B_6 are.

Normal daily recommended intakes for pyridoxine are generally defined as follows:

- Infants and children—
  Birth to 3 years of age: 0.3 to 1 milligram (mg).
  4 to 6 years of age: 1.1 mg.
  7 to 10 years of age: 1.4 mg.
- Adolescent and adult males—1.7 to 2 mg.
- Adolescent and adult females—1.4 to 1.6 mg.
- Pregnant females—2.2 mg.
- Breast-feeding females—2.1 mg.

Before Using This Dietary Supplement

If you are taking this dietary supplement without a prescription, carefully read and follow any precautions on the label. For pyridoxine, the following should be considered:

Pregnancy—Excessive doses of pyridoxine taken during pregnancy may cause the infant to become dependent on pyridoxine.

Medicines or other dietary supplements— Although certain medicines or dietary supplements should not be used together at all, in other cases they may be used together even if an interaction might occur. In these cases, your health care professional may want to change the dose, or other precautions may be necessary. When you are taking pyridoxine, it is especially important that your health care professional know if you are taking the following:

- Levodopa (e.g., Larodopa)—Use with pyridoxine may prevent the levodopa from working properly

---

Proper Use of This Dietary Supplement

To use the *extended-release capsule form* of this dietary supplement:

- Swallow the capsule whole.
- Do not crush, break, or chew before swallowing.
- If the capsule is too large to swallow, you may mix the contents of the capsule with jam or jelly and swallow without chewing.

To use the *extended-release tablet form* of this dietary supplement:

- Swallow the tablet whole.
- Do not crush, break, or chew before swallowing.

Side Effects of This Dietary Supplement

Along with its needed effects, a dietary supplement may cause some unwanted effects. Although pyridoxine does not usually cause any side effects at usual doses, check with your health care professional as soon as possible if you notice either of the following side effects:

With large doses
   Clumsiness; numbness of hands or feet

Also check with your health care professional if you notice any other unusual effects while you are taking pyridoxine.

Other Claimed Uses

Claims that pyridoxine is effective for treatment of acne and other skin problems, alcohol intoxication, asthma, hemorrhoids, kidney stones, mental problems, migraine headaches, morning sickness, and menstrual problems, or to stimulate appetite or milk production have not been proven.

RIBOFLAVIN
(Vitamin B₂)   Systemic

Generic name product is available in the U.S. and Canada.

Description

Vitamins (VYE-ta-mins) are compounds that you *must* have for growth and health. They are needed in small amounts only and are usually available in the foods that you eat. Riboflavin (RYE-boe-flay-vin) (vitamin B_2) is needed for metabolism of carbohydrates, proteins, and fats. It also makes it possible for oxygen to reach your cells.

Lack of riboflavin may lead to itching and burning eyes, sensitivity of eyes to light, sore tongue, itching and peeling skin on the nose and scrotum, and sores in the mouth. Your health care professional may treat this condition by prescribing riboflavin for you.

Some conditions may increase your need for riboflavin. These include:

- Alcoholism
- Burns
- Cancer
- Diarrhea (continuing)
- Fever (continuing)
- Illness (continuing)

- Infection
- Intestinal diseases
- Liver disease
- Overactive thyroid
- Serious injury
- Stress (continuing)
- Surgical removal of stomach

In addition, riboflavin may be given to infants with high blood levels of bilirubin (hyperbili-rubinemia).

Increased need for riboflavin should be determined by your health care professional.

Riboflavin is available without a prescription in the following dosage form:

Oral
- Tablets (U.S. and Canada)

Importance of Diet

Riboflavin is found in various foods, including milk and dairy products, fish, meats, green leafy vegetables, and whole grain and enriched cereals and bread. Food processing may destroy some of the vitamins, although little riboflavin is lost from foods during ordinary cooking.

Normal daily recommended intakes in milligrams (mg) for riboflavin are generally defined as follows:

Persons	U.S. (mg)	Canada (mg)
Infants and children		
Birth to 3 years of age	0.4–0.8	0.3–0.7
4 to 6 years of age	1.1	0.9
7 to 10 years of age	1.2	1–1.3
Adolescent and adult males	1.4–1.8	1–1.6
Adolescent and adult females	1.2–1.3	1–1.1
Pregnant females	1.6	1.1–1.4
Breast-feeding females	1.7–1.8	1.4–1.5

Side Effects of This Dietary Supplement

Along with its needed effects, a dietary supplement may cause some unwanted effects. Riboflavin may cause urine to have a more yellow color than normal, especially if large doses are taken. This is to be expected and is no cause for alarm. Usually, however, riboflavin does not cause any side effects. Check with your health care professional if you notice any other unusual effects while you are using it.

Other Claimed Uses

Claims that riboflavin is effective for treatment of acne, some kinds of anemia (weak blood), migraine headaches, and muscle cramps have not been proven.

SELENIUM SUPPLEMENTS   Systemic

Some commonly used brand names are:

In the U.S.—
   Sele-Pak[1]
   Selepen[1]

Note: For quick reference, the following selenium supplements are numbered to match the corresponding brand names.

This information applies to the following:

1. Selenious Acid (se-LEE-nee-us as-id)†‡
2. Selenium (se-LEE-nee-um)‡§

---

†Not commercially available in Canada.

‡Generic name product may also be available in the U.S.

§Generic name product may also be available in Canada.

Description

Selenium supplements are used to prevent or treat selenium deficiency.

The body needs selenium for normal growth and health. Selenium is needed for certain enzymes that help with normal body functions.

Lack of selenium may lead to changes in fingernails, muscle weakness, and heart problems.

Selenium deficiency in the United States is rare. Patients receiving total parenteral nutrition (TPN) for long periods of time may need selenium. Selenium deficiency is a problem in areas of the world where the soil contains little selenium.

Injectable selenium is administered only by or under the supervision of your health care professional. Another form of selenium is available without a prescription.

Selenium supplements are available in the following dosage forms:

 Oral
  Selenium
   • Tablets (U.S. and Canada)
 Parenteral
  Selenious Acid
   • Injection (U.S.)

Importance of Diet

Selenium is found in seafood, liver, lean red meat, and grains grown in soil that is rich in selenium.

Normal daily recommended intakes for selenium are generally defined as follows:

• Infants and children—
 Birth to 3 years of age: 10 to 20 micrograms (mcg).
 4 to 6 years of age: 20 mcg.
 7 to 10 years of age: 30 mcg.
• Adolescent and adult males—40 to 70 mcg.
• Adolescent and adult females—45 to 55 mcg.

- Pregnant females—65 mcg.
- Breast-feeding females—75 mcg.

Side Effects of This Dietary Supplement

Along with its needed effects, a dietary supplement may cause some unwanted effects. Although selenium supplements have not been reported to cause any side effects, check with your health care professional immediately if any of the following side effects occur as a result of an overdose:

Symptoms of overdose

> Diarrhea; fingernail weakening; garlic odor of breath and sweat; hair loss; irritability; itching of skin; metallic taste; nausea and vomiting; unusual tiredness and weakness

Other side effects not listed above may also occur in some individuals. If you notice any other effects, check with your health care professional.

Other Claimed Uses

Although selenium is being used to prevent certain types of cancer, there is not enough information to show that this is effective.

SODIUM FLUORIDE   Systemic

Some commonly used brand names are:

In the U.S.—

Fluoritab	Luride Lozi-Tabs
Fluorodex	Luride-SF Lozi-Tabs
Flura	Pediaflor
Flura-Drops	Pharmaflur
Flura-Loz	Pharmaflur 1.1
Karidium	Pharmaflur df
Luride	Phos-Flur

Generic name product may also be available.

In Canada—

Flozenges	Karidium
Fluor-A-Day	PDF
Fluoritabs	Pedi-Dent
Fluorosol	Solu-Flur

Generic name product may also be available.

Description

Fluoride has been found to be helpful in reducing the number of cavities in the teeth. It is usually present naturally in drinking water. However, some areas of the country do not have a high enough level in the water to prevent cavities. To make up for this, extra fluorides may be added to the diet. Some children may require both dietary fluorides and topical fluoride treatments by the dentist. Use of a fluoride toothpaste or rinse may be helpful as well.

Taking fluorides does not replace good dental habits. These include eating a good diet, brushing and flossing teeth often, and having regular dental checkups.

Sodium fluoride is available only with a prescription, in the following dosage forms:

Oral

- Lozenges (U.S. and Canada)
- Oral solution (U.S. and Canada)
- Tablets (U.S. and Canada)
- Chewable tablets (U.S. and Canada)

Importance of Diet

People get needed fluoride from fish, including the bones, tea, and drinking water that has fluoride added to it. Food that is cooked in water containing fluoride or in Teflon-coated pans also provides fluoride. However, foods cooked in aluminum pans provide less fluoride.

Normal daily recommended intakes for fluoride are generally defined as follows:

- Infants and children—
  Birth to 3 years of age: 0.1 to 1.5 milligrams (mg).
  4 to 6 years of age: 1 to 2.5 mg.
  7 to 10 years of age: 1.5 to 2.5 mg.
- Adolescents and adults—1.5 to 4 mg.

Remember:

- The total amount of fluoride you get every day includes what you get from the foods and beverages that you consume and what you may take as a supplement.
- This total amount *should not* be greater than the above recommendations, unless

ordered by your health care professional. Taking too much fluoride can cause serious problems to the teeth and bones.

Before Using Sodium Fluoride

In deciding to use sodium fluoride, the risks of taking it must be weighed against the good it will do. This is a decision you and your health care professional will make. For sodium fluoride, the following should be considered:

Pregnancy—Sodium fluoride occurs naturally in water and has not been shown to cause problems in infants of mothers who drank fluoridated water or took appropriate doses of supplements.

Children—Doses of sodium fluoride that are too large or are taken for a long time may cause bone problems and teeth discoloration in children.

Older adults—Older people are more likely to have joint pain, kidney problems, or stomach ulcers which may be made worse by taking large doses of sodium fluoride. You should check with your health care professional.

Other medical problems—The presence of other medical problems may affect the use of sodium fluoride. Make sure you tell your health care professional if you have any other medical problems, especially:

- Brown, white, or black discoloration of teeth or
- Joint pain or
- Kidney problems (severe) or
- Stomach ulcer—Sodium fluoride may make these conditions worse

---

Proper Use of Sodium Fluoride

Take sodium fluoride only as directed by your health care professional. Do not take more of it and do not take it more often than ordered. Taking too much fluoride over a period of time may cause unwanted effects.

For individuals taking the *chewable tablet form* of sodium fluoride:

- Tablets should be chewed or crushed before they are swallowed.
- Sodium fluoride works best if it is taken at bedtime, after the teeth have been thoroughly brushed. Do not eat or drink for at least 15 minutes after taking sodium fluoride.

For individuals taking the *oral liquid form* of this sodium fluoride:

- Sodium fluoride is to be taken by mouth even though it comes in a dropper bottle. The amount to be taken is to be measured with the specially marked dropper.
- *Always store sodium fluoride in the original plastic container.* Fluoride will affect glass and should not be stored in glass containers.

- Sodium fluoride may be dropped directly into the mouth or mixed with cereal, fruit juice, or other food. However, if sodium fluoride is mixed with foods or beverages that contain calcium, the amount of sodium fluoride that is absorbed may be reduced.

Precautions While Using Sodium Fluoride

The level of fluoride present in the water is different in different parts of the U.S. If you move to another area, check with a health care professional in the new area as soon as possible to see if sodium fluoride is still needed or if the dose needs to be changed. Also, check with your health care professional if you change infant feeding habits (e.g., breast-feeding to infant formula), drinking water (e.g., city water to nonfluoridated bottled water), or filtration (e.g., tap water to filtered tap water).

Do not take calcium supplements or aluminum hydroxide–containing products and sodium fluoride at the same time. It is best to space doses of these two products 2 hours apart, to get the full benefit from each.

Inform your health care professional as soon as possible if you notice white, brown, or black spots on the teeth. These are signs of too much fluoride in children when it is given during periods of tooth development.

Side Effects of Sodium Fluoride

Along with its needed effects, sodium fluoride may cause some unwanted effects. Although not all of these side effects may occur, if they do occur they may need medical attention.

Check with your health care professional as soon as possible if the following side effect occurs:

Sores in mouth and on lips (rare)

Sodium fluoride in drinking water or taken as a supplement does not usually cause any side effects. However, *taking an overdose of fluoride may cause serious problems.*

Stop taking sodium fluoride and check with your health care professional immediately if any of the following side effects occur, as they may be symptoms of severe overdose:

Black, tarry stools; bloody vomit; diarrhea; drowsiness; faintness; increased watering of mouth; nausea or vomiting; shallow breathing; stomach cramps or pain; tremors; unusual excitement; watery eyes; weakness

Check with your health care professional as soon as possible if the following side effects occur, as some may be early symptoms of possible chronic overdose:

Pain and aching of bones; stiffness; white, brown, or black discoloration of teeth—occurs only during periods of tooth development in children

Other side effects not listed above may also occur in some individuals. If you notice any other effects, check with your health care professional.

SODIUM IODIDE Systemic†

A commonly used brand name in the U.S. is Iodopen.
Generic name product may also be available.

†Not commercially available in Canada.

Description

Sodium iodide (SOE-dee-um EYE-oh-died) is used to prevent or treat iodine deficiency.

The body needs iodine for normal growth and health. For patients who are unable to get enough iodine in their regular diet or who have a need for more iodine, sodium iodide may be necessary. Iodine is needed so that your thyroid gland can function properly.

Iodine deficiency in the United States is rare because iodine is added to table salt. Most people get enough salt from the foods they eat, without adding salt to their meals. Iodine deficiency is a problem in other areas of the world.

Lack of iodine may lead to thyroid problems, mental problems, hearing loss, and goiter.

Sodium iodide is available by itself only as an injection, which is administered by or under the supervision of your health care professional. Some multivitamin/mineral preparations that contain sodium iodide are available without a prescription.

Sodium iodide is available in the following dosage forms:

Oral

Sodium Iodide
Sodium iodide is available orally as part of a multivitamin/mineral combination.

Parenteral

Sodium Iodide
• Injection (U.S.)

Importance of Diet

Iodine is found in various foods, including seafood, small amounts of iodized salt, and vegetables grown in iodine-rich soils. Iodine-containing mist from the ocean is another important source of iodine, since iodine is absorbed by the skin. Iodized salt provides 76 micrograms (mcg) of iodine per gram of salt.

Normal daily recommended intakes in micrograms (mcg) for iodine are generally defined as follows:

Persons	U.S. (mcg)	Canada (mcg)
Infants and children		
Birth to 3 years of age	40–70	30–65
4 to 6 years of age	90	85
7 to 10 years of age	120	95–125
Adolescent and adult males	150	125–160
Adolescent and adult females	150	110–160
Pregnant females	175	135–185
Breast-feeding females	200	160–210

Before Using This Dietary Supplement

If you are taking this dietary supplement without a prescription, carefully read and follow any precautions on the label. For sodium iodide, the following should be considered:

Pregnancy—A deficiency of iodine in the mother may cause nerve or growth problems for the fetus. Taking high doses of sodium iodide may cause thyroid problems or goiter in the newborn infant.

Breast-feeding—Taking high doses of sodium iodide while breast-feeding may cause skin rash and thyroid problems in nursing babies.

Children—Taking high doses of sodium iodide may cause skin rash and thyroid problems in infants.

Medicines or other dietary supplements— Although certain medicines or dietary supplements should not be used together at all, in other cases they may be used together even if an interaction might occur. In these cases, your health care professional may want to change the dose, or other precautions may be necessary. When you are taking sodium iodide, it is especially important that your health care professional know if you are taking any of the following:

- Antithyroid agents (medicine for overactive thyroid)—These medicines may prevent sodium iodide from working properly
- Iodine-containing preparations, other—Use of these preparations with sodium iodide may

increase blood levels of iodine, which may increase the chance of side effects
- Lithium (e.g., Lithane)—Use of this medicine with sodium iodide may increase the chance of side effects

Other medical problems—The presence of other medical problems may affect the use of sodium iodide. Make sure you tell your health care professional if you have any other medical problems, especially:
- Kidney disease—Use of sodium iodide may increase the amount of iodine in the blood and increase the chance of side effects
- Thyroid disease—This condition may increase the chance of side effects of sodium iodide
- Tuberculosis—Use of sodium iodide may make this condition worse

Precautions While Using This Dietary Supplement

Many other products contain iodine. For example, iodine is absorbed through the skin from some skin cleansers (e.g., povidone-iodine). It may be especially important that infants and small children not receive large amounts of iodine. Check with your health care professional before using any other products that contain iodine while you are using sodium iodide.

Side Effects of This Dietary Supplement

Along with its needed effects, a dietary supplement may cause some unwanted effects.

Although not all of these side effects may occur, if they do occur they may need medical attention. When this dietary supplement is used at low doses, side effects are rare.

Check with your health care professional as soon as possible if any of the following side effects occur:

Less common

Hives; joint pain; swelling of arms, face, legs, lips, tongue, and/or throat; swelling of lymph glands

With long-term use

Burning of mouth or throat; headache (severe); increased watering of mouth; metallic taste; skin sores; soreness of teeth and gums; stomach irritation

Other side effects not listed above may also occur in some individuals. If you notice any other effects, check with your health care professional.

THIAMINE
(Vitamin B₁) Systemic

Some commonly used brand names are:

In the U.S.—
Biamine

Generic name product may also be available.

In Canada—
Betaxin   Bewon

Generic name product may also be available.

Description

Vitamins (VYE-ta-mins) are compounds that you *must* have for growth and health. They are needed in small amounts only and are usually available in the foods that you eat. Thiamine (THYE-a-min) (vitamin B₁) is needed in the breakdown of carbohydrates.

Some conditions may increase your need for thiamine. These include:

- Alcoholism
- Burns
- Diarrhea (continuing)
- Fever (continuing)
- Illness (continuing)
- Intestinal diseases
- Liver disease
- Overactive thyroid
- Stress (continuing)
- Surgical removal of stomach

Also, the following groups of people may have a deficiency of thiamine:

- Patients using an artificial kidney (on hemodialysis)
- Individuals who do heavy manual labor on a daily basis

Increased need for thiamine should be determined by your health care professional.

Lack of thiamine may lead to a condition called beriberi. Signs of beriberi include loss of appetite, constipation, muscle weakness, pain or tingling in arms or legs, and possible swelling of feet or lower legs. In addition, if severe, lack of thiamine may cause mental depression, memory problems, weakness, shortness of breath, and fast heartbeat. Your health care professional may treat this by prescribing thiamine for you.

Injectable thiamine is administered only by or under the supervision of your health care professional. Other forms of thiamine are available without a prescription.

Thiamine is available in the following dosage forms:

Oral
- Elixir (Canada)
- Tablets (U.S. and Canada)

Parenteral
- Injection (U.S. and Canada)

Importance of Diet

Thiamine is found in various foods, including cereals (whole-grain and enriched), peas, beans, nuts, and meats (especially pork and beef). Some thiamine in foods is lost with cooking.

Normal daily recommended intakes in milligrams (mg) for thiamine are generally defined as follows:

Persons	U.S. (mg)	Canada (mg)
Infants and children		
Birth to 3 years of age	0.3–0.7	0.3–0.6
4 to 6 years of age	0.9	0.7
7 to 10 years	1	0.8–1
Adolescent and adult males	1.2–1.5	0.8–1.3
Adolescent and adult females	1–1.1	0.8–0.9
Pregnant females	1.5	0.9–1
Breast-feeding females	1.6	1–1.1

Side Effects of This Dietary Supplement
Along with its needed effects, a dietary supplement may cause some unwanted effects. Although not all of these side effects may occur, if they do occur they may need medical attention.

Check with your health care professional immediately if any of the following side effects occur:
Rare—Soon after receiving injection only
Coughing; difficulty in swallowing; hives; itching of skin; swelling of face, lips, or eyelids; wheezing or difficulty in breathing

Other side effects not listed above may also occur in some individuals. If you notice any other effects, check with your health care professional.

Other Claimed Uses

Claims that thiamine is effective for treatment of skin problems, chronic diarrhea, tiredness, mental problems, multiple sclerosis, nerve problems, and ulcerative colitis (a disease of the intestines), as an insect repellant or to stimulate appetite have not been proven.

VITAMIN A Systemic

A commonly used brand name in the U.S. and Canada is Aquasol A.

Another commonly used name is retinol.

Generic name product may also be available in the U.S. and Canada.

Description

Vitamins (VYE-ta-mins) are compounds that you *must* have for growth and health. They are needed in small amounts only and are usually available in the foods that you eat. Vitamin A is needed for night vision and for growth of skin, bones, and male and female reproductive organs. In pregnant women vitamin A is necessary for the growth of a healthy fetus.

Lack of vitamin A may lead to a rare condition called night blindness (problems seeing in the dark), as well as dry eyes, eye infections, skin problems, and slowed growth. Your health care professional may treat these problems by prescribing vitamin A for you.

Some conditions may increase your need for vitamin A. These include:

- Diarrhea
- Eye diseases
- Intestinal diseases
- Infections (continuing or chronic)

- Measles
- Pancreas disease
- Stomach removal
- Stress (continuing)

In addition, infants receiving unfortified formula may need vitamin A supplements.

Vitamin A absorption will be decreased in any condition in which fat is poorly absorbed.

Increased need for vitamin A should be determined by your health care professional.

Injectable vitamin A is administered only by or under the supervision of your health care professional. Other forms of vitamin A are available without a prescription.

Vitamin A is available in the following dosage forms:

Oral
- Capsules (U.S. and Canada)
- Oral solution (U.S.)
- Tablets (U.S.)

Parenteral
- Injection (U.S.)

Importance of Diet

Vitamin A is found in various foods, including yellow-orange fruits and vegetables; dark green, leafy vegetables; vitamin A–fortified milk; liver; and margarine. Vitamin A comes in two different forms, retinols and beta-carotene. Retinols are found in foods that come from animals (meat, milk, eggs). The form of vitamin A found in plants is called beta-carotene (which is converted to vitamin A in the body). Food processing may destroy some of the vitamins. For example, freezing may reduce the amount of vitamin A in foods.

In the past, the recommended intakes for vitamin A have been expressed in Units. This term Units has been replaced by retinol equivalents (RE) or micrograms (mcg) of retinol, with 1 RE equal to 1 mcg of retinol. This was done to better describe the two forms of vitamin A, retinol and beta-carotene. One RE of vitamin A is equal to 3.33 Units of retinol and 10 Units of beta-carotene. Some products available have not changed their labels and continue to be labeled in Units.

Normal daily recommended intakes in the United States for vitamin A are generally defined according to age or condition and to the form of vitamin A as follows:

Age or Condition	Form of Vitamin A		
	RE or mcg of Retinol	Amount in Units as Retinol	Amount in Units as a Combination of Retinol and Beta-carotene*
Infants and children			
Birth to 3 years	375–400	1250–1330	1875–2000
4 to 6 years	500	1665	2500
7 to 10 years	700	2330	3500
Adolescent and adult males	1000	3330	5000
Adolescent and adult females	800	2665	4000
Pregnant females	800	2665	4000
Breast-feeding females	1200–1300	4000–4330	6000–6500

*Based on 1980 recommended dietary allowances (RDAs) for vitamin A in the diet that is a combination of retinol and beta-carotene.

Normal daily recommended intakes in Canada for vitamin A are generally defined according to age or condition and to the form of vitamin A as follows:

Age or Condition	Form of Vitamin A		
	RE or mcg of Retinol	Amount in Units as Retinol	Amount in Units as a Combination of Retinol and Beta-carotene*
Infants and children			
Birth to 3 years	400	1330	2000
4 to 6 years	500	1665	2500
7 to 10 years	700–800	2330–2665	3500
Adolescent and adult males	1000	3330	5000
Adolescent and adult females	800	2665	4000
Pregnant females	900	2665–3000	4000–4500
Breast-feeding females	1200	4000	6000

*Based on 1980 U.S. recommended dietary allowances (RDAs) for vitamin A in the diet that is a combination of retinol and beta-carotene.

Before Using This Dietary Supplement
If you are taking this dietary supplement
without a prescription, carefully read and follow any precautions on the label. For vitamin
A, the following should be considered:

Pregnancy—Taking too much vitamin A
(more than 1800 RE [6000 Units]) during pregnancy can cause harmful effects such as birth
defects or slow or reduced growth in the
child.

Children—Side effects from high doses and/
or prolonged use of vitamin A are more likely
to occur in young children than adults.

Older adults—Some studies have shown that
the elderly may be at risk of high blood levels
of vitamin A with long-term use.

Dental—High doses and/or prolonged use of
vitamin A may cause bleeding from the gums;
dry or sore mouth; or drying, cracking, or
peeling of the lips.

Medicines or other dietary supplements—
Although certain medicines or dietary supplements should not be used together at all, in
other cases they may be used together even
if an interaction might occur. In these cases,
your health care professional may want to
change the dose, or other precautions may be
necessary. When you are taking vitamin A, it
is especially important that your health care
professional know if you are taking any of
the following:

- Etretinate or
- Isotretinoin (e.g., Accutane)—Use with vitamin A may cause high blood levels of vitamin A, which may increase the chance of side effects

Other medical problems—The presence of other medical problems may affect the use of vitamin A. Make sure you tell your health care professional if you have any other medical problems, especially:

- Alcohol abuse (or history of) or
- Liver disease—Vitamin A use may make liver problems worse
- Kidney disease—May cause high blood levels of vitamin A, which may increase the chance of side effects

---

Proper Use of This Dietary Supplement

For individuals taking the *oral liquid form* of vitamin A:

- This preparation is to be taken by mouth even though it comes in a dropper bottle.
- This dietary supplement may be dropped directly into the mouth or mixed with cereal, fruit juice, or other food.

Precautions While Using This Dietary Supplement

Vitamin A is stored in the body; therefore, when you take more than the body needs, it

will build up in the body. This may lead to
poisoning and even death. Problems are more
likely to occur in:

- Adults taking 7500 RE (25,000 Units) a
  day for 8 months in a row, or 450,000 RE
  (1,500,000 Units) all at once; or
- Children taking 5400 RE (18,000 Units) to
  15,000 RE (50,000 Units) a day for several
  months in a row, or 22,500 RE (75,000
  Units) to 105,100 RE (350,000 Units) all
  at once.
- Pregnant women taking more than 1800
  RE (6000 Units) a day.

Remember that the total amount of vitamin A
you get every day includes what you get from
foods that you eat and what you take as a
supplement.

Side Effects of This Dietary Supplement

Along with its needed effects, a dietary supplement may cause some unwanted effects.
Vitamin A does not usually cause any side
effects at normal recommended doses. *However, taking large amounts of vitamin A over a
period of time may cause some unwanted effects
that can be serious. Check with your health care
professional immediately* if any of the following
side effects occur, since they may be signs of
sudden overdose:

Bleeding from gums or sore mouth; bulging soft
  spot on head (in babies); confusion or unusual excitement; diarrhea; dizziness or

drowsiness; double vision; headache (severe); irritability (severe); peeling of skin, especially on lips and palms; vomiting (severe)

Check with your health care professional as soon as possible if any of the following side effects occur, since they may also be signs of gradual overdose:

Bone or joint pain; convulsions (seizures); drying or cracking of skin or lips; dry mouth; fever; general feeling of discomfort or illness or weakness; headache; increased sensitivity of skin to sunlight; increase in frequency of urination, especially at night, or in amount of urine; irritability; loss of appetite; loss of hair; stomach pain; unusual tiredness; vomiting; yellow-orange patches on soles of feet, palms of hands, or skin around nose and lips

Other side effects not listed above may also occur in some individuals. If you notice any other effects, check with your health care professional.

Other Claimed Uses

Claims that vitamin A is effective for treatment of conditions such as acne or lung diseases, or for treatment of eye problems, wounds, or dry or wrinkled skin not caused by lack of vitamin A have not been proven. Although vitamin A is being used to prevent certain types of cancer, some experts feel there is not enough information to show that this is effective, particularly in well-nourished individuals.

VITAMIN B₁₂ Systemic

Some commonly used brand names are:

In the U.S.—

Alphamin[2]	Hydroxy-Cobal[2]
Cobex[1]	LA-12[2]
Cobolin-M[1]	Neuroforte-R[1]
Crystamine[1]	Primabalt[1]
Crysti-12[1]	Rubesol-1000[1]
Cyanoject[1]	Rubramin PC[1]
Cyomin[1]	Shovite[1]
Hydrobexan[2]	Vibal[1]
Hydro-Cobex[2]	Vibal LA[2]
Hydro-Crysti-12[2]	Vitabee 12[1]

In Canada—
Anacobin[1]
Bedoz[1]

Note: For quick reference, the following supplements are numbered to match the corresponding brand names.

This information applies to the following:

1. Cyanocobalamin (sye-an-oh-koe-BAL-a-min)‡
2. Hydroxocobalamin (hye-drox-oh-koe-BAL-a-min)†‡

---

†Not commercially available in Canada.

‡Generic name product may also be available in the U.S.

Description

Vitamins (VYE-ta-mins) are compounds that you *must* have for growth and health. They are needed in small amounts only and are usually available in the foods that you eat. Vitamin B₁₂ is necessary for healthy blood. Cyanocobalamin and hydroxocobalamin are man-made forms of vitamin B₁₂.

Some people have a medical problem called pernicious anemia in which vitamin B$_{12}$ is not absorbed from the intestine. Others may have a badly diseased intestine or have had a large part of their stomach or intestine removed, so that vitamin B$_{12}$ cannot be absorbed. These people need to receive vitamin B$_{12}$ by injection.

Some conditions may increase your need for vitamin B$_{12}$. These include:

- Alcoholism
- Anemia, hemolytic
- Fever (continuing)
- Genetic disorders such as homocystinuria and/or methylmalonic aciduria
- Intestinal diseases
- Infections (continuing or chronic)
- Kidney disease
- Liver disease
- Pancreas disease
- Stomach disease
- Stress (continuing)
- Thyroid disease
- Worm infections

In addition, persons who are strict vegetarians or follow macrobiotic diets may need vitamin B$_{12}$ supplements.

Increased need for vitamin B$_{12}$ supplements should be determined by your health care professional.

Lack of vitamin B$_{12}$ may lead to anemia (weak blood), stomach problems, and nerve damage. Your health care professional may treat this by prescribing vitamin B$_{12}$ for you.

Injectable vitamin B$_{12}$ is administered only by or under the supervision of your health care professional. Some strengths of oral vitamin B$_{12}$ are available only with your health care professional's prescription. Others are available without a prescription.

Vitamin B$_{12}$ is available in the following dosage forms:

Oral

Cyanocobalamin
- Extended-release tablets (U.S.)
- Tablets (U.S. and Canada)

Parenteral

Cyanocobalamin
- Injection (U.S. and Canada)

Hydroxocobalamin
- Injection (U.S.)

Importance of Diet

Vitamin B$_{12}$ is found in various foods, including fish, egg yolk, milk, and fermented cheeses. It is *not* found in any vegetables. Ordinary cooking probably does not destroy the vitamin B$_{12}$ in food.

Normal daily recommended intakes in micrograms (mcg) for vitamin B$_{12}$ are generally defined as follows:

Persons	U.S. (mcg)	Canada (mcg)
Infants and children		
Birth to 3 years of age	0.3–0.7	0.3–0.4
4 to 6 years of age	1	0.5
7 to 10 years of age	1.4	0.8–1
Adolescent and adult males	2	1–2
Adolescent and adult females	2	1–2
Pregnant females	2.2	2–3
Breast-feeding females	2.6	1.5–2.5

Before Using This Dietary Supplement

If you are taking this dietary supplement without a prescription, carefully read and follow any precautions on the label. For vitamin B₁₂, the following should be considered:

Pregnancy—You may need vitamin B₁₂ supplements if you are a strict vegetarian (vegan-vegetarian) or follow a macrobiotic diet. Too little vitamin B₁₂ can cause harmful effects such as anemia or nervous system injury.

Breast-feeding—If you are a strict vegetarian or follow a macrobiotic diet, your baby may not be getting the vitamin B₁₂ needed.

Other medical problems—The presence of other medical problems may affect the use of vitamin B₁₂. Make sure you tell your health care professional if you have any other medical problems, especially:

- Leber's disease (an eye disease)—Vitamin B₁₂ may make this condition worse

Proper Use of This Dietary Supplement

For patients receiving vitamin B$_{12}$ by injection for pernicious anemia or if part of the stomach or intestine has been removed:

- You will have to receive treatment for the rest of your life. You must continue to receive vitamin B$_{12}$ even if you feel well, in order to prevent future problems.

Side Effects of This Dietary Supplement

Along with its needed effects, a dietary supplement may cause some unwanted effects. Cyanocobalamin or hydroxocobalamin do not usually cause any side effects. *However, check with your health care professional immediately* if any of the following side effects occur:

Rare—soon after receiving injection only

Skin rash or itching; wheezing

Check with your health care professional as soon as possible if either of the following side effects continues or is bothersome:

Less common

Diarrhea; itching of skin

Other side effects not listed above may also occur in some individuals. If you notice any other effects, check with your health care professional.

Other Claimed Uses

Claims that vitamin B$_{12}$ is effective for treatment of various conditions such as aging, allergies, eye problems, slow growth, poor appetite or malnutrition, skin problems, tiredness, mental problems, sterility, thyroid disease, and nerve diseases have not been proven. Many of these treatments involve large and expensive amounts of vitamins.

VITAMIN D and Related Compounds Systemic

Some commonly used brand names are:

In the U.S.—

Calciferol[5]	DHT Intensol[4]
Calciferol Drops[5]	Drisdol[5]
Calcijex[3]	Drisdol Drops[5]
Calderol[2]	Hytakerol[4]
DHT[4]	Rocaltrol[3]

In Canada—

Calciferol[5]	One-Alpha[1]
Calcijex[3]	Ostoforte[5]
Drisdol[5]	Radiostol Forte[5]
Hytakerol[4]	Rocaltrol[3]

Note: For quick reference, the following vitamin D and related compounds are numbered to match the corresponding brand names.

This information applies to the following:

1. Alfacalcidol (al-fa-KAL-si-dol)*
2. Calcifediol (kal-si-fe-DYE-ole)†
3. Calcitriol (kal-si-TRYE-ole)
4. Dihydrotachysterol (dye-hye-droh-tak-ISS-ter-ole)
5. Ergocalciferol (er-goe-kal-SIF-e-role)‡§

---

*Not commercially available in the U.S.
†Not commercially available in Canada.
‡Generic name product may also be available in the U.S.
§Generic name product may also be available in Canada.

Description

Vitamins (VYE-ta-mins) are compounds that you *must* have for growth and health. They are needed in small amounts only and are available in the foods that you eat. Vitamin D helps your body absorb calcium. It is necessary for strong bones and teeth.

Lack of vitamin D may lead to a condition called rickets, especially in children, in which bones and teeth are weak. In adults it may cause a condition called osteomalacia, in which calcium is lost from bones so that they become weak. Your health care professional may treat these problems by prescribing vitamin D for you. Vitamin D is also sometimes used to treat other diseases in which calcium is not used properly by the body.

Ergocalciferol is the form of vitamin D used in vitamin supplements.

Some conditions may increase your need for vitamin D. These include:
- Alcoholism
- Intestinal diseases
- Kidney disease
- Liver disease
- Pancreas disease
- Surgical removal of stomach

In addition, individuals and breast-fed infants who lack exposure to sunlight, those who follow a strict vegetarian or macrobiotic diet, as well as dark-skinned individuals, may be more likely to have a vitamin D deficiency.

Increased need for vitamin D should be determined by your health care professional.

Alfacalcidol, calcifediol, calcitriol, and dihydrotachysterol are forms of vitamin D used to treat hypocalcemia (not enough calcium in the blood).

Injectable calcitriol and ergocalciferol are administered only by or under the supervision of your health care professional. Some strengths of oral ergocalciferol and all strengths of alfacalcidol, calcifediol, calcitriol, and dihydrotachysterol are available only with a prescription. Other strengths of oral ergocalciferol are available without a prescription. *Taking large amounts of vitamin D over long periods may cause serious unwanted effects.*

Vitamin D and related compounds are available in the following dosage forms:

Oral

Alfacalcidol
- Capsules (Canada)
- Oral solution (Canada)

Calcifediol
- Capsules (U.S.)

Calcitriol
- Capsules (U.S. and Canada)
- Oral solution (Canada)

Dihydrotachysterol
- Capsules (U.S. and Canada)
- Oral solution (U.S.)
- Tablets (U.S.)

Ergocalciferol
- Capsules (U.S. and Canada)
- Oral solution (U.S. and Canada)
- Tablets (U.S. and Canada)

Parenteral

Calcitriol
- Injection (U.S. and Canada)

Ergocalciferol
• Injection (U.S. and Canada)

Importance of Diet

Vitamin D is found naturally only in fish and fish-liver oils. However, it is also found in milk (vitamin D–fortified). Cooking does not affect the vitamin D in foods. Vitamin D is sometimes called the "sunshine vitamin," since it is made in your skin when you are exposed to sunlight. If you eat a balanced diet and get outside in the sunshine at least 1.5 to 2 hours a week, you should be getting all the vitamin D you need.

In the past, the Recommended Dietary Allowances (RDAs) and Recommended Nutrient Intakes (RNIs) for vitamin D have been expressed in Units. This term has been replaced by micrograms (mcg) of vitamin D. Some manufacturers continue to label their products in Units.

Normal daily recommended intakes in mcg and Units are generally defined as follows:

Persons	U.S.		Canada	
	(mcg)	Units	(mcg)	Units
Infants and children				
Birth to 3 years of age	7.5–10	300–400	5–10	200–400
4 to 6 years of age	10	400	5	200
7 to 10 years of age	10	400	2.5–5	100–200

Persons	U.S.		Canada	
	(mcg)	Units	(mcg)	Units
Adolescent and adult males	5–10	200–400	2.5–5	100–200
Adolescent and adult females	5–10	200–400	2.5–5	100–200
Pregnant females	10	400	5–7.5	200–300
Breast-feeding females	10	400	5–7.5	200–300

Before Using This Dietary Supplement

If you are taking this dietary supplement without a prescription, carefully read and follow any precautions on the label. For vitamin D and related compounds, the following should be considered:

Pregnancy—You may need vitamin D supplements if you are a strict vegetarian (vegan-vegetarian) and/or have little exposure to sunlight and do not drink vitamin D–fortified milk.

Taking too much alfacalcidol, calcifediol, calcitriol, dihydrotachysterol, or ergocalciferol can also be harmful to the fetus. Taking more than your health care professional has recommended can cause your baby to be more sensitive than usual to its effects, can cause problems with a gland called the parathyroid, and can cause a defect in the baby's heart.

Breast-feeding—Infants who are totally breast-fed and have little exposure to the sun may require vitamin D supplementation. Your health care professional may recommend that you give your baby a vitamin supplement that contains vitamin D.

Children—Some studies have shown that infants who are totally breast-fed, especially with dark-skinned mothers, and have little exposure to sunlight may be at risk of vitamin D deficiency. Your health care professional may prescribe a vitamin/mineral supplement that contains vitamin D. Some infants may be sensitive to even small amounts of alfacalcidol, calcifediol, calcitriol, dihydrotachysterol, or ergocalciferol. Also, children may show slowed growth when receiving large doses of alfacalcidol, calcifediol, calcitriol, dihydrotachysterol, or ergocalciferol for a long time.

Older adults—Studies have shown that older adults may have lower blood levels of vitamin D than younger adults, especially those who have little exposure to sunlight. Your health care professional may recommend that you take a vitamin supplement that contains vitamin D.

Medicines or other dietary supplements—Although certain medicines or dietary supplements should not be used together at all, in other cases they may be used together even if an interaction might occur. In these cases, your health care professional may want to change the dose, or other precautions may be necessary. When you are taking vitamin D and related compounds it is especially important that your health care professional know if you are taking any of the following:

- Antacids containing magnesium—Use of these products with any vitamin D–related compound may result in high blood levels of magnesium, especially in patients with kidney disease
- Calcium-containing preparations or
- Thiazide diuretics (water pills)—Use of these medicines with vitamin D may cause high blood levels of calcium and increase the chance of side effects
- Vitamin D and related compounds, other—Use of vitamin D with a related compound may cause high blood levels of vitamin D and increase the chance of side effects

Other medical problems—The presence of other medical problems may affect the use of vitamin D and related compounds. Make sure you tell your health care professional if you have any other medical problems, especially:

- Heart or blood vessel disease—Alfacalcidol, calcifediol, calcitriol, or dihydrotachysterol may cause hypercalcemia (high blood levels of calcium), which may make these conditions worse
- Kidney disease—High blood levels of alfacalcidol, calcifediol, calcitriol, dihydrotachysterol, or ergocalciferol may result, which may increase the chance of side effects
- Sarcoidosis—May increase sensitivity to alfacalcidol, calcifediol, calcitriol, dihydrotachysterol, or ergocalciferol and increase the chance of side effects

Proper Use of This Dietary Supplement

For individuals taking the *oral liquid form* of this dietary supplement:

- This preparation should be taken by mouth even though it comes in a dropper bottle.
- This dietary supplement may be dropped directly into the mouth or mixed with cereal, fruit juice, or other food.

While you are taking alfacalcidol, calcifediol, calcitriol, or dihydrotachysterol, your health care professional may want you to follow a special diet or take a calcium supplement. Be sure to follow instructions carefully. If you are already taking a calcium supplement or any medicine containing calcium, make sure your health care professional knows.

Precautions While Using This Dietary Supplement

Vitamin D is stored in the body. *Taking large amounts over a period of time may cause some unwanted effects that can be serious.*

Do not take any nonprescription (over-the-counter [OTC]) medicine or dietary supplement that contains calcium, phosphorus, or vitamin D while you are taking any of these dietary supplements unless you have been told to do so by your health care professional. The extra calcium, phosphorus, or vitamin D may increase the chance of side effects.

Do not take antacids or other medicines containing magnesium while you are taking vitamin D. Taking vitamin D with these medicines may cause unwanted effects.

Side Effects of This Dietary Supplement

Along with its needed effects, a dietary supplement may cause some unwanted effects. Alfacalcidol, calcifediol, calcitriol, dihydrotachysterol, and ergocalciferol do not usually cause any side effects when taken as directed.

Check with your health care professional immediately if any of the following effects occur:

Late symptoms of severe overdose

High blood pressure; irregular heartbeat; stomach pain (severe)

Check with your health care professional as soon as possible if any of the following effects occur:

Early symptoms of overdose

Constipation (especially in children or adolescents); diarrhea; dryness of mouth; headache (continuing); increased thirst; increase in frequency of urination, especially at night, or in amount of urine; loss of appetite; metallic taste; nausea or vomiting (especially in children or adolescents); unusual tiredness or weakness

Late symptoms of overdose

Bone pain; cloudy urine; drowsiness; increased sensitivity of eyes to light or irritation of eyes; itching of skin; mood or

mental changes; muscle pain; nausea or
vomiting; weight loss

Other side effects not listed above may also
occur in some individuals. If you notice any
other effects, check with your health care
professional.

Other Claimed Uses

Claims that vitamin D is effective for treatment of arthritis and prevention of nearsight-
edness or nerve problems have not been
proven. Some psoriasis patients may benefit
from vitamin D supplements; however, con-
trolled studies have not been performed.

VITAMIN E   Systemic

Some commonly used brand names are:

In the U.S.—

Amino-Opti-E	E-400 I.U. in a Water
Aquasol E	Soluble Base
E-Complex-600	E-Vitamin Succinate
E-200 I.U. Softgels	Liqui-E
E-1000 I.U. Softgels	Pheryl-E
	Vita Plus E

Generic name product may also be available.

In Canada—

Aquasol E	Webber Vitamin E

Generic name product may also be available.

Another commonly used name is alpha tocopherol.

Description

Vitamins (VYE-ta-mins) are compounds that you *must* have for growth and health. They are needed in only small amounts and are available in the foods that you eat. Vitamin E prevents a chemical reaction called oxidation, which can sometimes result in harmful effects in your body. It is also important for the proper function of nerves and muscles.

Lack of vitamin E is extremely rare, except in people who have a disease in which it is not absorbed into the body.

Some conditions may increase your need for vitamin E. These include:

- Intestinal disease
- Liver disease

- Pancreas disease
- Surgical removal of stomach

In addition, infants who are receiving a formula that is not fortified with vitamin E may be likely to have a vitamin E deficiency. Also, diets high in polyunsaturated fatty acids may increase your need for vitamin E.

Increased need for vitamin E should be determined by your health care professional.

Vitamin E is available without a prescription in the following dosage forms:

Oral

- Capsules (U.S. and Canada)
- Oral solution (U.S. and Canada)
- Tablets (U.S.)
- Chewable tablets (U.S.)

Importance of Diet

Vitamin E is found in various foods including vegetable oils (corn, cottonseed, soybean, safflower), wheat germ, whole-grain cereals, and green leafy vegetables. Cooking and storage may destroy some of the vitamin E in foods.

Vitamin E is available in various forms, including *d*- or *dl*-alpha tocopheryl acetate, *d*- or *dl*-alpha tocopherol, and *d*- or *dl*-alpha tocopheryl acid succinate. In the past, the Recommended Dietary Allowances (U.S.) and Recommended Nutrient Intakes (Canada) for vitamin E have been expressed in Units. This term has been replaced by alpha tocopherol

equivalents (alpha-TE) or milligrams (mg) of
d-alpha tocopherol. One Unit is equivalent to
1 mg of *dl*-alpha tocopherol acetate or 0.6 mg
d-alpha tocopherol. Most products available
in stores continue to be labeled in Units.

Normal daily recommended intakes in milligrams of *d*-alpha tocopherol (mg alpha-TE)
and Units for vitamin E are generally defined
as follows:

Persons	U.S.		Canada	
	mg alpha-TE	Units	mg alpha-TE	Units
Infants and children				
Birth to 3 years of age	3–6	5–10	3–4	5–6.7
4 to 6 years of age	7	11.7	5	8.3
7 to 10 years of age	7	11.7	6–8	10–13
Adolescent and adult males	10	16.7	6–10	10–16.7
Adolescent and adult females	8	13	5–7	8.3–11.7
Pregnant females	10	16.7	8–9	13–15
Breast-feeding females	11–12	18–20	9–10	15–16.7

Before Using This Dietary Supplement

If you are taking this dietary supplement
without a prescription, carefully read and follow any precautions on the label. For vitamin
E, the following should be considered:

Children—You should check with your
health care professional if you are giving your
baby an unfortified formula. In that case, the
baby must get the vitamins needed some
other way. Some studies have shown that premature infants may have low levels of vitamin E. Your health care professional may
recommend a vitamin E supplement.

Other medical problems—The presence of
other medical problems may affect the use of
vitamin E. Make sure you tell your health care
professional if you have any other medical
problems, especially:

- Bleeding problems—Vitamin E in doses
  greater than 800 Units a day for prolonged
  periods may make this condition worse

Proper Use of This Dietary Supplement

For individuals taking the *oral liquid form of
this dietary supplement:*

- This preparation should be taken by
  mouth even though it comes in a dropper bottle.
- This dietary supplement may be
  dropped directly into the mouth or
  mixed with cereal, fruit juice, or other
  food.

Side Effects of This Dietary Supplement

Along with its needed effects, a dietary supplement may cause some unwanted effects.

When used for short periods of time at recommended doses, vitamin E usually does not cause any side effects. However, check with your health care professional as soon as possible if any of the following side effects occur:

With doses greater than 400 Units a day and long-term use

> Blurred vision; diarrhea; dizziness; headache; nausea or stomach cramps; unusual tiredness or weakness

Other side effects not listed above may also occur in some individuals. If you notice any other effects, check with your health care professional.

Other Claimed Uses

Claims that vitamin E is effective for treatment of cancer and for prevention or treatment of acne, aging, loss of hair, bee stings, liver spots on the hands, bursitis, diaper rash, frostbite, stomach ulcer, heart attacks, labor pains, certain blood diseases, miscarriage, muscular dystrophy, poor posture, sexual impotence, sterility, infertility, menopause, sunburn, and lung damage from air pollution have not been proven.

Vitamin E and Cancer

Claimed use: Some people think that taking vitamin E supplements may be useful in reducing the risk of cancer.

Possible action: Vitamin E may reduce the risk of cancer by protecting the body from unstable molecules known as free radicals. Free radicals are molecules that result from natural body processes. It is believed that by a process called oxidation, free radicals damage the body's cells. This is thought to be one of the many possible causes of cancer. As an antioxidant, vitamin E binds to free radicals and makes them inactive.

Current findings: The results from two major studies have become available over the past few years. One study involved 30,000 adults in Linxian, China. After five years, the group receiving daily supplements of beta-carotene (15 milligrams [mg]), vitamin E (30 mg [50 Units]), and selenium (50 micrograms [mcg]) had a lower rate of cancer, especially stomach cancer. Another study of 29,000 male smokers in Finland found no reduction in the incidence of lung cancer in the group receiving 50 mg (83 Units) of vitamin E a day for five to eight years.

Role of diet: The recommended daily intake of vitamin E is approximately 15 to 20 Units. This is far less than the amount needed to reduce the risk of cancer in the Linxian, China, study. It would be difficult to get that amount of vitamin E, 50 Units, from your diet alone.

Conclusion: The Linxian study took place in an area of China where a high rate of malnutrition and stomach cancer exists. For this reason, many researchers are not ready to assume that vitamin E prevents cancer in the U.S. In addition, three supplements with antioxidant properties (beta-carotene, selenium, and vitamin E) were taken together, making it difficult to separate out any one as having a positive influence by itself. Results from several large studies over the next few years should help determine the role of vitamin E in the prevention of cancer.

Additional reading: The Linxian, China, study can be found in the *Journal of the National Cancer Institute*, 1993, Volume 85, pages 1483-92. The Finnish study can be found in the *New England Journal of Medicine*, 1994, Volume 330, pages 1029-35. Additional information on vitamin E can be found in the following publication: *Consumer Reports on Health*, April 1993, pages 33-36.

Vitamin E and Heart Disease

Claimed use: Some people think that taking vitamin E supplements may help reduce the risk of heart disease.

Possible action: Vitamin E is one of several vitamins known as antioxidants. It is thought that vitamin E may reduce the risk of heart disease by preventing the oxidation (thus antioxidant) of low-density lipoprotein (LDL). LDL carries the bad cholesterol in the blood. Oxidation of LDL causes plaque buildup, which eventually clogs the arteries. This is only one of the many factors that cause heart disease.

Current findings: Researchers have reported some evidence that vitamin E supplements may reduce the risk of heart disease. The researchers collected information on the intake of vitamin E from 87,000 female nurses and 46,000 male health professionals. Intake from both diet and supplements was included. The results indicate that those subjects who chose to take vitamin E supplements (amounts of approximately 100 Units or more) had about a one-third lower risk of heart disease.

Role of diet: The recommended daily intake of vitamin E is approximately 15 to 20 Units. This is far less than the amount needed to reduce the risk of heart disease in the two studies. It would be difficult to get that amount, 100 Units, of vitamin E from your diet alone.

Conclusion: It is possible that other factors also helped to lower the risk of heart disease in the vitamin E takers in these studies. Therefore, the researchers point out that recommendations for widespread use of vitamin E supplements should await the results of additional studies. Results from several studies in which a large number of people are given vitamin E supplements should be available over the next few years.

Additional reading: The two studies mentioned above can be found in the *New England Journal of Medicine*, 1993, volume 328, pages 1340-1346 and 1444-1449. Additional information on vitamin E can be found in the following publications: *Consumer Reports on Health*, April 1993, pages 33-36; *Nutrition Action Healthletter*, January/February 1993, pages 8-11.

VITAMIN K Systemic

Some commonly used brand names are:

In the U.S.—
AquaMEPHYTON[2]   Mephyton[2]
Konakion[2]   Synkayvite[1]

Note: For quick reference, the following are numbered to match the corresponding brand names.

Another commonly used name is phytomenadione.

This information applies to the following:

1. Menadiol (men-a-DYE-ole)†
2. Phytonadione (fye-toe-na-DYE-one)§

---

†Not commercially available in Canada.

§Generic name product may also be available in Canada.

Description

Vitamins (VYE-ta-mins) are compounds that you *must* have for growth and health. They are needed in only small amounts and are usually available in the foods that you eat. Vitamin K is necessary for normal clotting of the blood. Vitamin K is routinely given to newborn infants to prevent bleeding problems.

Lack of vitamin K is rare but may lead to problems with blood clotting and increased bleeding. Your doctor may treat this by prescribing vitamin K for you.

Vitamin K is available without a prescription as part of some multivitamin/mineral combination products. Vitamin K is available only with a prescription, in the following dosage forms:

Oral

Menadiol
  • Tablets (U.S.)
Phytonadione
  • Tablets (U.S.)

Parenteral

Menadiol
  • Injection (U.S.)
Phytonadione
  • Injection (U.S. and Canada)

Importance of Diet

Vitamin K is found in various foods including green leafy vegetables, meat, and dairy products. If you eat a balanced diet containing these foods, you should be getting all the vitamin K you need. Little vitamin K is lost from foods with ordinary cooking.

Normal daily recommended intakes are generally defined as follows:

• Infants and children—
  Birth to 3 years of age: 5–15 micrograms (mcg).
  4 to 6 years of age: 20 mcg.
  7 to 10 years of age: 30 mcg.
• Adolescent and adult males—45–80 mcg.
• Adolescent and adult females—45–65 mcg.
• Pregnant females—65 mcg.
• Breast-feeding females—65 mcg.

Before Using Vitamin K

In deciding to use vitamin K, the risks of taking it must be weighed against the good it will do. This is a decision you and your doctor will make. For vitamin K, the following should be considered:

Breast-feeding—You should check with your doctor if you are giving your baby an unfortified formula. In that case, the baby must get the vitamins needed some other way.

Children—Children may be especially sensitive to the effects of vitamin K, especially menadiol. This may increase the chance of side effects during treatment.

Other medicines—Although certain medicines and vitamin K should not be used together at all, in other cases they may be used together even if an interaction might occur. In these cases, your doctor may want to change the dose, or other precautions may be necessary. When you are taking vitamin K, it is especially important that your health care professional know if you are taking any of the following:

- Acetohydroxamic acid (e.g., Lithostat) or
- Antidiabetics, oral (diabetes medicine you take by mouth) or
- Dapsone or
- Furazolidone (e.g., Furoxone) or
- Methyldopa (e.g., Aldomet) or
- Nitrofurantoin (e.g., Furadantin) or
- Primaquine or
- Procainamide (e.g., Pronestyl) or

- Quinidine (e.g., Quinidex) or
- Quinine (e.g., Quinamm) or
- Sulfonamides (sulfa medicine) or
- Sulfoxone (e.g., Diasone)—The chance of a serious side effect may be increased, especially with menadiol
- Anticoagulants (blood thinners)—Vitamin K decreases the effects of these medicines and is sometimes used to treat bleeding caused by anticoagulants; however, anyone receiving an anticoagulant should not take any supplement that contains vitamin K (alone or in combination with other vitamins or nutrients) unless it has been ordered by their doctor

Other medical problems—The presence of other medical problems may affect the use of vitamin K. Make sure you tell your doctor if you have any other medical problems, especially:

- Cystic fibrosis or
- Diarrhea (prolonged) or
- Intestinal problems—These conditions may interfere with absorption of vitamin K into the body when it is taken by mouth; higher doses may be needed, or the vitamin K may have to be injected
- Glucose-6-phosphate dehydrogenase (G6PD) deficiency or
- Liver disease—The chance of unwanted effects may be increased

---

Proper Use of Vitamin K

Take vitamin K only as directed by your doctor. Do not take more or less of it, do not take it more often, and do not take it for a longer time than your doctor ordered. To do so may cause serious unwanted effects such as blood clotting problems.

Your doctor should check your progress at regular visits. A blood test must be taken regularly to see how fast your blood is clotting. This will help your doctor decide how much vitamin K you need.

Missed dose—If you miss a dose of vitamin K, take it as soon as possible. However, if it is almost time for your next dose, skip the missed dose and go back to your regular dosing schedule. Do not double doses. *Tell your doctor about any doses you miss.*

Precautions While Using Vitamin K

Tell all health care professionals you go to that you are taking vitamin K.

Always check with your health care professional before you start or stop taking any other medicine. This includes any nonprescription (over-the-counter [OTC]) medicine, even aspirin. Other medicines may change the way vitamin K affects your body.

Side Effects of Vitamin K

Along with its needed effects, vitamin K may cause some unwanted effects. Although vitamin K does not usually cause side effects that need medical attention, check with your health care professional if any of the following side effects continue or are bothersome:

Less common

Flushing of face; redness, pain, or swelling at place of injection; unusual taste

Other side effects not listed above may also occur in some patients. If you notice any other effects, check with your health care professional.

ZINC SUPPLEMENTS Systemic

Some commonly used brand names are:

In the U.S.—

Orazinc[3]	Zinc-220[3]
Verazinc[3]	Zinca-Pak[3]
Zinc 15[3]	Zincate[3]

In Canada—
PMS Egozinc[3]

Note: For quick reference, the following zinc supplements are numbered to match the corresponding brand names.

This information applies to the following:

1. Zinc Chloride (zink KLOR-ide)[†‡]
2. Zinc Gluconate (GLOO-coh-nate)[‡§]
3. Zinc Sulfate (SUL-fate)[‡]

[†]Not commercially available in Canada.

[‡]Generic name product may also be available in the U.S.

[§]Generic name product may also be available in Canada.

Description

Zinc supplements are used to prevent or treat zinc deficiency.

The body needs zinc for normal growth and health. For patients who are unable to get enough zinc in their regular diet or who have a need for more zinc, zinc supplements may be necessary. They are generally taken by mouth but some patients may have to receive them by injection.

Lack of zinc may lead to poor night vision and wound-healing, a decrease in the sense of taste and smell, a reduced ability to fight infections, and poor development of reproductive organs.

Some conditions may increase your need for zinc. These include:

- Acrodermatitis enteropathica (a lack of absorption of zinc from the intestine)
- Alcoholism
- Burns
- Diabetes mellitus (sugar diabetes)
- Down's syndrome
- Eating disorders
- Intestinal diseases
- Infections (continuing or chronic)
- Kidney disease
- Liver disease
- Pancreas disease
- Sickle cell disease
- Skin disorders
- Stomach removal
- Stress (continuing)
- Thalassemia
- Trauma (prolonged)

In addition, premature infants may need additional zinc.

Increased need for zinc should be determined by your health care professional.

Injectable zinc is administered only by or under the supervision of your health care professional. Other forms of zinc are available without a prescription.

Zinc supplements are available in the following dosage forms:

Oral

Zinc Gluconate
- Lozenges (U.S.)
- Tablets (U.S. and Canada)

Zinc Sulfate
- Capsules (U.S.)
- Tablets (U.S. and Canada)
- Extended-release tablets (U.S.)

Parenteral

Zinc Chloride
- Injection (U.S.)

Zinc Sulfate
- Injection (U.S.)

Importance of Diet

Zinc is found in various foods, including lean red meats, seafoods (especially herring and oysters), peas, and beans. Zinc is also found in whole grains; however, large amounts of whole grains have been found to decrease the amount of zinc that is absorbed. Additional zinc may be added to the diet through treated (galvanized) cookware. Foods stored in uncoated tin cans may cause less zinc to be available for absorption from food.

Normal daily recommended intakes in milligrams (mg) for zinc are generally defined as follows:

Persons	U.S. (mg)	Canada (mg)
Infants and children		
Birth to 3 years of age	5–10	2–4
4 to 6 years of age	10	5
7 to 10 years of age	10	7–9
Adolescent and adult males	15	9–12
Adolescent and adult females	12	9
Pregnant females	15	15
Breast-feeding females	16–19	15

Before Using This Dietary Supplement

If you are taking this dietary supplement without a prescription, carefully read and follow any precautions on the label. For zinc supplements, the following should be considered:

Pregnancy—There is evidence that low blood levels of zinc may lead to problems in pregnancy or defects in the baby. Check with your health care professional.

Older adults—There is some evidence that the elderly may be at risk of becoming deficient in zinc due to poor food selection, decreased absorption of zinc by the body, or medicines that decrease absorption of zinc or increase loss of zinc from the body.

Medicines or other dietary supplements—Although certain medicines or dietary supplements should not be used together at all, in other cases they may be used together even if an interaction might occur. In these cases, your health care professional may want to change the dose, or other precautions may be necessary. When you are taking zinc supplements, it is especially important that your health care professional know if you are taking any of the following:

- Copper supplements or
- Tetracycline (taken by mouth) (medicine for infection)—Use with zinc supplements may cause copper supplements or tetracycline to be less effective; zinc supplements should be given at least 2 hours before or after copper supplements or tetracycline

Other medical problems—The presence of other medical problems may affect the use of zinc supplements. Make sure you tell your health care professional if you have any other medical problems, especially:

- Copper deficiency—Zinc supplements may make this condition worse

---

Precautions While Using This Dietary Supplement

When zinc combines with certain foods it may not be absorbed into your body and it will do you no good. If you are taking zinc, the following foods should be avoided or taken 2 hours after you take zinc:

- Bran
- Fiber-containing foods
- Phosphorus-containing foods such as milk or poultry
- Whole-grain breads and cereals

Do not take zinc supplements and copper, iron, or phosphorus supplements at the same time. It is best to space doses of these products 2 hours apart, to get the full benefit from each dietary supplement.

Side Effects of This Dietary Supplement

Along with its needed effects, a dietary supplement may cause some unwanted effects. Although not all of these side effects may occur, if they do occur, they may need medical attention.

Check with your health care professional as soon as possible if any of the following side effects occur:

Rare—With large doses

Chills; continuing ulcers or sores in mouth or throat; fever; heartburn; indigestion; nausea; sore throat; unusual tiredness or weakness

Symptoms of overdose

Chest pain; dizziness; fainting; shortness of breath; vomiting; yellow eyes or skin

Other side effects not listed above may also occur in some individuals. If you notice any other effects, check with your health care professional.

Other Claimed Uses

Claims that zinc is effective in preventing vision loss in the elderly have not been proven. Zinc has not been proven effective in the treatment of porphyria.

GLOSSARY

Abdomen—The body area between the chest and pelvis.

Abortifacient—Medicine that causes abortion.

Abrade—Scrape or rub away the outer cover or layer of a part.

Absorption—Passing into the body; incorporation of substances into or across tissues of the body, for example, digested food into the blood from the small intestine, or poisons through the skin.

Achlorhydria—Absence of acid that normally would be found in the stomach.

Acidifier, urinary—Medicine that makes the urine more acidic.

Acidosis—Too much acidity or loss of alkalinity in the body fluids and tissues.

Acromegaly—Enlargement of the face, hands, and feet because of too much growth hormone.

Acute—Sharp or intense; describes a condition that begins suddenly, has severe symptoms, and usually lasts a short time.

Added fiber—In food labeling, at least 2.5 grams of more fiber per serving than reference food.

Addison's disease—Disease caused by not enough secretion of corticosteroid hormones by the adrenal glands; causes weakness, salt loss, and low blood pressure.

Adhesion—The union by connective tissue of

two parts that are normally separate (such as parts of a joint).

Adjunct—An additional or secondary treatment that is helpful but is not necessary to treatment of a particular condition; not effective for that condition if used alone.

Adjuvant—1. A substance added to or used with another substance to assist its action. 2. Something that assists or enhances the effectiveness of medical treatment.

Adrenal cortex—Outer layer of tissue of the adrenal gland, which produces corticosteroid hormones.

Adrenal glands—Two organs located next to the kidneys. They produce the hormones epinephrine and norepinephrine and corticosteroid hormones, such as cortisol.

Adrenaline—See epinephrine.

Adrenal medulla—Inner part of the adrenal gland, which produces epinephrine and norepinephrine.

Adrenocorticoids—See Corticosteroids.

Aerosol—Suspension of very small liquid or solid particles in compressed gas; drugs in aerosol form are dispensed in the form of a mist by releasing the gas.

African sleeping sickness—See Trypanosomiasis, African.

Agent—A force or substance capable of causing a change.

Agoraphobia—Fear of public places or open spaces.

Agranulocytosis—Disorder in which there is

a severe decrease in the number of granulocytes normally present in the blood.

AIDS (acquired immunodeficiency syndrome)—Disease caused by human immunodeficiency virus (HIV). The disease results in a breakdown of the body's immune system, which makes a person more likely to get some other infections and some forms of cancer.

Alcohol-abuse deterrent—Medicine used to help alcoholics avoid the use of alcohol.

Alkaline—Having a pH of more than 7. Opposite of acidic.

Alkalizer, urinary—Medicine that makes the urine more alkaline.

Alkalosis—Too much alkalinity or loss of acidity in the body fluids and tissues.

Alopecia—Loss or absence of hair from areas where it normally is present; baldness.

Altitude sickness agent—Medicine used to prevent or lessen some of the effects of high altitude on the body.

Alzheimer's disease—Progressive disorder of thinking and other mental processes, usually beginning in late middle age.

Aminoglycosides—A class of chemically related antibiotics used to treat some serious types of bacterial infections.

Anabolic steroids—Synthetic forms of male hormones.

Analgesic—Medicine that relieves pain without causing unconsciousness.

Anaphylaxis—Sudden, severe allergic reaction.

Androgen—Substance, such as testosterone, that stimulates development of male characteristics.

Anemia—Reduction, to below normal, of hemoglobin in the blood.

Anesthesiologist—A physician who is qualified to give an anesthetic and other medicines to a patient before and during surgery.

Anesthetic—Medicine that causes a loss of feeling or sensation, especially of pain, sometimes through loss of consciousness.

Aneurysm—Abnormal dilatation or saclike swelling of an artery, vein, or the heart.

Angina—Pain, tightness, or feeling of heaviness in the chest, due mostly to lack of oxygen for the heart muscle. The pain may be felt in the left shoulder, jaw, or arm instead of or in addition to the chest. Symptoms often occur during exercise.

Angioedema—Allergic condition marked by continuing swelling and severe itching of areas of the skin.

Anorexia—Loss of appetite for food.

Anoxia—Absence of oxygen. The term is sometimes incorrectly used for hypoxia, which means an abnormally low amount of oxygen in the body.

Antacid—Medicine used to neutralize excess acid in the stomach.

Antagonist—Drug or other substance that blocks or works against the action of another.

Anthelmintic—Medicine used to destroy or expel intestinal worms.

Antiacne agent—Medicine used to treat acne.

Antianemic—Agent that prevents or corrects anemia.

Antianginal—Medicine used to prevent or treat angina attacks.

Antianxiety agent—Medicine used to treat excessive nervousness, tension, or anxiety.

Antiarrhythmic—Medicine used to treat irregular heartbeats.

Antiasthmatic—Medicine used to treat asthma.

Antibacterial—Medicine that kills or stops the growth of bacteria.

Antibiotic—Chemical substance used to treat infections.

Antibody—Special kind of blood protein that helps the body fight infection.

Antibulimic—Medicine used to treat bulimia.

Anticholelithic—Medicine used to dissolve gallstones.

Anticoagulant—Medicine used to prevent formation of blood clots in the blood vessels.

Anticonvulsant—Medicine used to prevent or treat convulsions (seizures).

Antidepressant—Medicine used to treat mental depression.

Antidiabetic agent—Medicine used to control blood sugar levels in patients with diabetes mellitus (sugar diabetes).

Antidiarrheal—Medicine used to treat diarrhea.

Antidiuretic—Medicine used to decrease formation of urine (for example, in patients with diabetes insipidus).

Antidote—Medicine used to prevent or treat harmful effects of another medicine or a poison.

Antidyskinetic—Medicine used to help treat the loss of muscle control caused by certain diseases or by some other medicines.

Antidysmenorrheal—Medicine used to treat menstrual cramps.

Antiemetic—Medicine used to prevent or treat nausea and vomiting.

Antiendometriotic—Medicine used to treat endometriosis.

Antienuretic—Medicine used to help prevent bedwetting.

Antifibrotic—Medicine used to treat fibrosis.

Antiflatulent—Medicine used to help relieve excess gas in the stomach or intestines.

Antifungal—Medicine used to treat infections caused by a fungus.

Antiglaucoma agent—Medicine used to treat glaucoma.

Antigout agent—Medicine used to prevent or relieve gout attacks.

Antihemorrhagic—Medicine used to prevent or help stop serious bleeding.

Antihistamine—Medicine used to prevent or relieve the symptoms of allergies (such as hay fever).

Antihypercalcemic—Medicine used to help lower the amount of calcium in the blood.

Antihyperlipidemic—Medicine used to help lower high levels of lipids in the blood.

Antihyperphosphatemic—Medicine used to help lower the amount of phosphate in the blood.

Antihypertensive—Medicine used to treat high blood pressure.

Antihyperuricemic—Medicine used to prevent or treat gout or other medical problems caused by too much uric acid in the blood.

Antihypocalcemic—Medicine used to increase calcium blood levels in patients with too little calcium.

Antihypoglycemic—Medicine used to increase blood sugar levels in patients with low blood sugar.

Antihypokalemic—Medicine used to increase potassium blood levels in patients with too little potassium.

Anti-infective—Medicine used to treat infection.

Anti-inflammatory—Medicine used to relieve pain, swelling, and other symptoms of inflammation.

Anti-inflammatory, nonsteroidal—An anti-inflammatory medicine that is not a cortisone-like medicine.

Anti-inflammatory, steroidal—A cortisone-like anti-inflammatory medicine.

Antimetabolite—Medicine that interferes with the normal processes within cells, preventing their growth.

Antimuscarinic—Medicine used to block the effects of a certain chemical in the body; often used to reduce smooth muscle spasms, especially abdominal or stomach cramps or spasms.

Antimyasthenic—Medicine used to treat myasthenia gravis.

Antimyotonic—Medicine used to prevent or relieve nighttime leg cramps or muscle spasms.

Antineoplastic—Medicine used to treat cancer.

Antineuralgic—Medicine used to treat neuralgia.

Antioxidant—Nutrient that protects tissues of the body against oxygen damage. The antioxidants are vitamins A, beta-carotene, C, and E.

Antiprotozoal—Medicine used to treat infections caused by protozoa.

Antipsoriatic—Medicine used to treat psoriasis.

Antipsychotic—Medicine used to treat certain nervous, mental, and emotional conditions.

Antipyretic—Medicine used to reduce fever.

Antirheumatic—Medicine used to treat arthritis (rheumatism).

Antirosacea—Medicine used to treat rosacea.

Antiseborrheic—Medicine used to treat dandruff and seborrhea.

Antiseptic—Medicine that stops the growth of germs. Used on the surface of the skin to prevent infections in cuts, scrapes, and wounds.

Antispasmodic—Medicine used to reduce smooth muscle spasms (for example, stomach, intestinal, or urinary tract spasms).

Antispastic—Medicine used to treat muscle spasms.

Antithyroid agent—Medicine used to treat an overactive thyroid gland.

Antitremor agent—Medicine used to treat tremors (trembling or shaking).

Antitubercular—Medicine used to treat tuberculosis (TB).

Antitussive—Medicine used to relieve cough.

Antiulcer agent—Medicine used to treat stomach and duodenal ulcers.

Antivertigo agent—Medicine used to prevent dizziness.

Antiviral—Medicine used to treat infections caused by a virus.

Anus—The opening at the end of the digestive tract through which bowel contents are passed.

Anxiety—An emotional state with apprehension, worry, or tension in reaction to real or imagined danger or dread of a situation; accompanied by sweating, increased pulse, trembling, weakness, and fatigue.

Apnea—Temporary absence of breathing.

Apoplexy—See Stroke.

Appendicitis—Inflammation of the appendix.

Appetite stimulant—Medicine used to help increase the desire for food.

Appetite suppressant—Medicine used in weight control programs to help decrease the desire for food.

Arrhythmia—Abnormal heart rhythm.

Arteritis, temporal—Inflammatory disease of arteries, usually of the head; occurs in older people.

Arthralgia—Pain in a joint.

Arthritis, rheumatoid—Chronic disease, especially of the joints, marked by pain and swelling.

Ascites—Accumulation of fluid in the abdominal cavity.

Asthma—Disease marked by inflammation of the bronchial tubes (air passages). During an attack, air passages become constricted, causing wheezing and difficult breathing. Attacks may be brought on by allergens, virus infection, cold air, or exercise.

Atherosclerosis—Common disease of the arteries in which artery walls thicken and harden.

Avoid—To keep away from deliberately.

Bacteremia—Presence of bacteria in the blood.

Bacterium—Tiny, one-celled organism. Different types of bacteria are responsible for a number of diseases and infections.

Bancroft's filariasis—Disease transmitted by mosquitos in which an infection with the filarial worm occurs. Affects the lymph system, producing inflammation.

Beriberi—Disorder caused by too little vitamin B$_1$ (thiamine), marked by an accumulation of fluid in the body, extreme weight loss, inflammation of nerves, or paralysis.

Bile—Thick fluid produced by the liver and stored in the gallbladder. Bile helps in the digestion of fats.

Bile duct—Tubular passage which carries bile from the liver to the gallbladder, or from the gallbladder to the intestine.

Bilharziasis—See Schistosomiasis.

Biliary—Relating to bile, the bile duct, or the gallbladder.

Bilirubin—The bile pigment that is orange-colored or yellow; an excess in the blood may cause jaundice.

Bipolar disorder—Severe mental illness marked by repeated episodes of depression and mania. Also called *manic-depressive illness.*

Bisexual—One who is sexually attracted to both sexes.

Black fever—See Leishmaniasis, visceral.

Blackwater fever—Condition, marked by dark urine, rarely seen as a complication of malaria.

Bone marrow—Soft material filling the cavities of bones.

Bone marrow depression—Condition in which the production of red blood cells, leukocytes, or platelets by the red bone marrow is decreased.

Bone resorption inhibitor—Medicine used to prevent or treat certain types of bone disorders, such as Paget's disease of the bone; helps prevent bone loss.

Bowel disease, inflammatory, suppressant—Medicine used to treat certain intestinal disorders, such as colitis.

Bradycardia—Slow heart rate, usually less than 60 beats per minute.

Bronchitis—Inflammation of the bronchial tubes (air passages) of the lungs.

Bronchodilator—Medicine used to open up the bronchial tubes (air passages) of the lungs to increase the flow of air through them.

Buccal—Relating to the cheek. A buccal medicine is taken by placing it in the pocket between the cheek and the gum and letting it slowly dissolve.

Bulimia—Disturbance in eating behavior marked by bouts of excessive eating followed by self-induced vomiting and diarrhea, hard exercise, or fasting.

Bursa—Small fluid-filled sac present where body parts move over one another (such as in a joint) to help reduce friction.

Bursitis—Inflammation of a bursa.

Calorie—Unit of heat that measures the energy value of food.

Calorie free—In food labeling, fewer than 5 calories per serving.

Candidiasis of the mouth—Overgrowth of the yeast *Candida* in the mouth marked by white patches on the tongue or inside the mouth. Also called *thrush* or *white mouth*.

Candidiasis of the vagina—Yeast infection of the vagina caused by the yeast *Candida;* associated with itching, burning, and a cheesy or curd-like white discharge.

Carbohydrate—Any one of a large group of compounds from plants, including sugars and starches, that contain only carbon, hydrogen, and oxygen. Carbohydrates are a source of energy for animals and humans.

Cardiac—Relating to the heart.

Cardiac arrhythmia—Irregularity or loss of the normal rhythm of the heartbeat.

Cardiac load–reducing agent—Medicine used to ease the workload of the heart by allowing the blood to flow through the blood vessels more easily.

Cardiotonic—Medicine used to improve the strength and efficiency of the heart.

Caries, dental—Tooth decay, sometimes causing pain, leading to the crumbling of the tooth. Also called *cavities*.

Cataract—An opacity (cloudiness) in the eye lens that impairs vision or causes blindness.

Catheter—Tube inserted into a small opening in the body so that fluids can be put in or taken out.

Caustic—Burning or corrosive agent; irritating and destructive to living tissue.

Cavity—1. Hollow space within the body. 2. Hole in a tooth, caused by dental caries.

Central nervous system—Part of the nervous system that is composed of the brain and spinal cord.

Cerebral palsy—Permanent disorder of motor weakness and loss of coordination due to damage to the brain.

Cervix—Lower end or necklike opening of the uterus to the vagina.

Chemotherapy—Treatment of illness or disease by chemical agents. The term most commonly refers to the use of drugs to treat cancer.

Chickenpox—See Varicella.

Chlamydia—A family of microorganisms that cause a variety of diseases in humans. One form is transmitted by sexual contact.

Cholesterol—Fatlike substance made by the liver but also absorbed from the diet; found only in animal tissues. Too much blood cholesterol is associated with several potential health risks, especially atherosclerosis (hardening of the arteries).

Cholesterol free—In food labeling, less than 2 milligrams of cholesterol and 2 grams or less of saturated fat per serving.

Chromosome—The structure in the cell nucleus that contains the DNA; in humans, there are normally 46.

Chronic—Describes a condition of long duration, which is often of gradual onset and may involve very slow changes. Note that

the term "chronic" has nothing to do with
how serious the condition is.

Cirrhosis—Chronic liver disease marked by
destruction of its cells and abnormal tissue growth.

Clitoris—Small, erectile body, being a part of
the female external sex organs.

CNS—See Central nervous system.

Cold sores—See Herpes simplex.

Colic—Waves of sudden severe abdominal
pain, which are usually separated by rela-
tively pain-free intervals.

Colitis—Inflammation of the colon (bowel).

Colony stimulating factor—Protein that stimulates the production of one or more kinds
of cells made in the bone marrow.

Colostomy—Operation in which part of the
colon (bowel) is brought through the abdominal wall to create an artificial opening.
The contents of the intestine are discharged
through the opening, bypassing the rest of
the intestines.

Coma—State of unconsciousness from which
the patient cannot be aroused.

Coma, hepatic—Disturbances in mental function and the nervous system caused by severe liver disease.

Condom—Thin sheath or cover worn over the
penis during sexual intercourse to prevent
pregnancy or infection; made of latex (rub-
ber) or animal intestine.

Congestive heart failure—Condition resulting from inability of the heart to pump

strongly enough to maintain adequate blood flow; characterized by breathlessness and edema.

Conjunctiva—Delicate mucous membrane covering the front of the eye and the inside of the eyelid.

Conjunctivitis—Inflammation of the conjunctiva.

Constriction—Squeezing together and becoming narrower or smaller, such as constriction of blood vessels or eye pupils.

Contagious disease—Disease that can be transmitted from one person to another.

Contamination—The introduction of germs or unclean material into or on normally sterile substances or objects.

Contraceptive—Medicine or device used to prevent pregnancy.

Contraction—A shortening or tightening, as in the normal function of muscles.

Convulsion—Sudden involuntary contraction or series of jerkings of muscles.

Corticosteroids—Group of cortisone-like hormones that are secreted by the adrenal cortex and are critical to the body. The two major groups of corticosteroids are glucocorticoids, which affect fat and body metabolism, and mineralocorticoids, which regulate salt/water balance. Also called *adrenocorticoids*.

Cortisol—Natural hormone produced by the adrenal cortex, important for carbohydrate, protein, and fat metabolism and for the normal response to stress; synthetic cortisol (hydrocortisone) is used to treat inflammations, allergies, collagen diseases, rheumatic disorders, and adrenal failure.

Cot death—See Sudden infant death syndrome (SIDS).

Cowpox—See Vaccinia.

Creutzfeldt-Jakob disease—Rare disease, probably caused by a slow-acting virus that affects the brain and nervous system.

Crib death—See Sudden infant death syndrome (SIDS).

Criteria—Standards on which a judgment or decision is based.

Crohn's disease—Chronic, inflammatory disease of the digestive tract, usually the lower small intestine.

Croup—Inflammation and blockage of the larynx (voice box) in young children.

Crystalluria—Crystals in the urine.

Cushing's syndrome—Condition in which the adrenal gland produces too much cortisone-like hormone, leading to weight gain, round face, and high blood pressure.

Cycloplegia—Paralysis of certain eye muscles; can be induced by medication for certain eye examinations.

Cycloplegic—Medicine used to induce cycloplegia.

Cyst—Abnormal sac or closed cavity filled with liquid or semisolid matter.

Cystic—Marked by cysts.

Cystic fibrosis—Hereditary disease of children and young adults which predominantly affects the lungs. Exocrine glands do not function normally, and excess mucus is produced.

Cystine—An amino acid found in most proteins; it is produced by the digestion of the protein.

Cystitis, interstitial—Inflammation of the bladder, predominantly in women, with frequent urge to urinate and painful urination.

Cytomegalovirus—One of a group of viruses. One form may be sexually transmitted and can be fatal in patients with weakened immune systems.

Cytoplasm—The contents of a cell outside the nucleus.

Cytotoxic agent—Chemical that kills cells or stops cell division; used to treat cancer.

Daily Value (DV)—Value used on food and dietary supplement labels to indicate the percent of the recommended daily amount of each nutrient that a serving provides. DV takes the place of USRDA (United States Recommended Daily Allowance).

Decongestant, nasal—Medicine used to help relieve nasal congestion (stuffy nose).

Decongestant, ophthalmic—Medicine used in the eye to relieve redness, burning, itching, or other irritation.

Decubitus—The position taken in lying down.

Decubitus ulcer—Bedsore; damage to the skin and underlying tissues caused by constant pressure.

Dental—Related to the teeth and gums.

Depression, mental—Condition marked by deep sadness; associated with lack of any pleasurable interest in life. Other symptoms include disturbances in sleep, appetite, and concentration, and difficulty in performing day-to-day tasks.

Dermatitis herpetiformis—Skin disease marked by sores and itching.

Dermatitis, seborrheic—Type of eczema found on the scalp and face.

Dermatomyositis—Inflammatory disorder of the skin and underlying tissues, including breakdown of muscle fibers.

Diabetes insipidus—Disorder in which the patient produces large amounts of dilute urine and is constantly thirsty. Also called *water diabetes*.

Diabetes mellitus—Disorder in which the body cannot process sugars to release energy; either the body does not produce enough insulin or the body tissues are unable to use the insulin present. This leads to too much sugar in the blood (hyperglycemia). Also called *sugar diabetes*.

Diagnose—Find out the cause or nature of a disorder by examination and laboratory tests.

Diagnostic procedure—A process carried out to determine the cause or nature of a condition, disease, or disorder.

Dialysis, renal—Artificial technique for removing waste materials or poisons from the blood when the kidneys are not working properly.

Digestant—Agent that will help in digestion.

Diplopia—Awareness of two images of a single object at one time; double vision.

Disintegration—The process of breaking down into small pieces. In nutrition, a measure of how fast a vitamin tablet or capsule breaks into small pieces in stomach fluids.

Dissolution—The breaking down of a substance into its separate parts. In nutrition, a measure of how fast a vitamin tablet or capsule dissolves once it has been swallowed.

Diuretic—Medicine used to increase the amount of urine produced by helping the kidneys get rid of water and salt. Also called *water pill.*

Diverticulitis—Inflammation of a diverticulum in the intestinal tract.

Diverticulum—Sac or pouch opening from a canal or cavity.

DNA—Deoxyribonucleic acid; the genetic material that controls heredity. DNA is located in the cell nucleus.

Down syndrome—Mental retardation associated with the presence of an extra chromosome 21. Patients with Down syndrome are marked physically by a round head, flat nose, slightly slanted eyes, and short stature. Also called *mongolism.*

Duct—Tube or channel, especially one that serves to carry secretions from a gland.

Dumdum fever—See Leishmaniasis, visceral.

Duodenal ulcer—Open sore in that part of the small intestine closest to the stomach.

Duodenum—First of the three parts of the small intestine.

Dyskinesia—Refers to abnormal, involuntary movement or a defect in voluntary movement.

Dyspnea—Shortness of breath; difficult breathing.

Eczema—Inflammation of the skin, marked by itching and rash.

Edema—Swelling of body tissue due to accumulation of fluids, usually first noticed in the feet or lower legs.

Eighth-cranial-nerve disease—Disease of the eighth cranial nerve, serving the inner ear; results in dizziness, loss of balance, loss of hearing, nausea, or vomiting.

Electrolyte—In medical use, chemicals (ions) in body fluids that are needed for normal functioning of the body. Body electrolytes include bicarbonate, chloride, sodium, potassium, etc.

Embolism—Sudden blocking of a blood vessel by a blood clot or foreign substances carried to the place of obstruction by the blood.

Embryo—In humans, a developing fertilized egg within the uterus (womb) from about two to eight weeks after fertilization.

Emergency—Extremely serious unexpected or sudden happening or situation that calls for immediate action.

Emollient—Substance that soothes and softens an irritated surface, such as the skin.

Emphysema—Lung condition in which destructive changes occur in the air spaces; air is not exchanged normally during the process of breathing in and out.

Encephalitis—Inflammation of the brain.

Encephalopathy—Any degenerative disease of the brain; caused by many different medical conditions.

Endocarditis—Inflammation of the lining of the heart, leading to fever, heart murmurs, and heart failure.

Endocrine gland—A gland that has no duct; releases its secretion directly into the blood.

Endometriosis—Condition in which material similar to the lining of the uterus (womb) appears at other sites within the pelvic cavity, causing pain and bleeding.

Enteric coating—Coating on tablets which allows them to pass through the stomach unchanged before being broken up in the intestine and being absorbed. Used to protect the stomach from the medicine and/or the medicine from the stomach's acid.

Enteritis—Inflammation of the small intestine, usually causing diarrhea.

Enuresis—Urinating while asleep (bedwetting).

Enzyme—Type of protein produced by cells

that may bring about or speed up a normal chemical reaction in the body.

Eosinophil—One type of white blood cells readily stained by the dye eosin; important in allergic reactions and parasitic infections.

Eosinophilia—Condition in which the number of eosinophils in the blood is abnormally high.

Epidural space—Area in the spinal column into which medicines (usually for pain) can be administered.

Epilepsy—Any of a group of brain disorders featuring sudden attacks of seizures and other symptoms.

Epinephrine—Hormone secreted by the adrenal medulla. It stimulates the heart, constricts blood vessels, and relaxes some smooth muscles. Also called *adrenaline*.

EPO—See Erythropoietin.

Ergot alkaloids—A class of medicines that cause narrowing of blood vessels; used to treat migraine headaches, and to reduce bleeding in childbirth.

Erythropoietin—Hormone secreted by the kidney. It controls the production of red blood cells by the bone marrow; also available as a synthetic drug (EPO).

Esophagus—The part of the digestive tract connecting the pharynx to the stomach.

Estrogen—Principal female sex hormone necessary for the normal sexual development of the female; during the menstrual cycle, its actions help prepare for possible pregnancy. Estrogen is often used to treat discomforts of menopause.

Exocrine gland—Any gland that discharges its secretion through a duct that opens on a surface (not into the blood).

Exophthalmos—Thrusting forward of the eyeballs in their sockets, giving the appearance of the eyes sticking out too far; commonly associated with hyperthyroidism.

Expectorant—Medicine used to help remove mucus or phlegm in the lungs by coughing or spitting it up.

Extrapyramidal symptoms—Movement disorders occurring with certain diseases or with use of certain drugs, including trembling and shaking of hands and fingers, twisting movements of the body, shuffling walk, and stiffness of arms or legs.

Familial Mediterranean fever—Inherited condition involving inflammation of the lining of the chest, abdomen, and joints. Also called *recurrent polyserositis*.

Fasciculation—Small, spontaneous contraction of a few muscle fibers, which is visible through the skin; muscular twitching.

Fat—An energy-rich organic compound that occurs naturally in animals and plants. Fats are an essential nutrient for humans.

Fat free—In food labeling, less than 0.5 grams of fat per serving.

Fatty acid—One of the basic organic compounds that make up lipids.

Favism—Inherited condition resulting from sensitivity to broad (fava) beans; marked by fever, vomiting, diarrhea, and acute destruction of red blood cells.

Fertility—Capacity to bring about the start of pregnancy.

Fertilization—Union of an ovum with a sperm.

Fetus—In humans, a developing baby within the uterus (womb) from about the beginning of the third month of pregnancy.

Fewer calories—In food labeling, at least 25 percent fewer calories per serving than the reference food.

Fiber—The carbohydrate material of food that cannot be digested. Fiber adds bulk to the diet.

Fibrocystic—Having benign (noncancerous) tumors of connective tissue.

Fibroid tumor—A noncancerous tumor of the uterus formed of fibrous or fully developed connective tissue.

Fibrosis—Condition in which the skin and underlying tissues tighten and become less flexible.

Fistula—Abnormal tubelike passage connecting two internal organs or one that leads from an abscess or internal organ to the body surface.

Flatulence—Excessive amount of air or gas in the stomach or intestine.

Flu—See Influenza.

Flushing—Temporary redness of the face and/or neck.

Food Guide Pyramid—An eating plan developed by Health and Human Services and the Department of Agriculture that describes the basic food groups. It serves as a guide for having a proper diet.

Fungus—Any of a group of simple organisms, including molds and yeasts.

Fungus infection—Infection caused by a fungus. Some common fungus infections are tinea pedis (athlete's foot), tinea capitis (ringworm of the scalp), tinea cruris (ringworm of the groin or jock itch), and mouth or vaginal candidiasis (yeast infections).

Gait—Manner of walk.

Gamma globulin—The portion of the blood that contains most of the antibodies associated with the body's immunity to infection.

Gastric—Relating to the stomach.

Gastric acid secretion inhibitor—Medicine used to decrease the amount of acid produced by the stomach.

Gastroenteritis—Inflammation of the stomach and intestine.

Gastroesophageal reflux—Backward flow into the esophagus of the contents of the stomach and duodenum. The condition is often characterized by "heartburn."

Generic—General in nature; relating to an entire group or class. In relation to medicines, the general name of a drug substance; not owned by one specific group as would be true for a trademark or brand name.

Genital—1. Relating to the organs concerned with reproduction; the sexual organs. 2. Relating to reproduction.

Genital warts—Small growths found on the genitals or around the anus; caused by a virus. The disease may be transmitted by sexual contact.

Gilles de la Tourette syndrome—See Tourette's disorder.

Gingiva—Gums.

Gingival hyperplasia—Overgrowth of the gums.

Gingivitis—Inflammation of the gums.

Glandular fever—See Mononucleosis.

Glaucoma—Condition of abnormally high pressure in the eye; may lead to loss of vision if not treated.

Glomeruli—Clusters of capillaries in the nephrons of the kidney that act as filters of the blood.

Glomerulonephritis—Inflammation of the glomeruli of the kidney not directly caused by infection.

Glucose-6-phosphate dehydrogenase (G6PD) deficiency—Lack of or reduced amounts of an enzyme (glucose-6-phosphate dehydrogenase) that helps the breakdown of certain sugar compounds in the body.

Gluten—Type of protein found primarily in wheat and rye.

Goiter—Enlargement of the thyroid gland that causes the neck to swell. Condition usually results from a lack of iodine or overactivity of the thyroid gland.

Gonadotropin—Any hormone that stimulates the activities of the ovaries or testes.

Gonorrhea—An infectious disease, usually transmitted by sexual contact. It causes infection in the genital organs in both men and women, and may also result in systemic disease.

Good source of fiber—In food labeling, 2.5 grams to 4.9 grams of fiber per serving.

Gout—Disease in which too much uric acid builds up in the blood and joints, leading to inflammation of the joints.

Granulation—Small, fleshy outgrowths on the healing surface of a wound or ulcer; a normal stage in healing.

Granulocyte—A class of white blood cell.

Granulocytopenia—Abnormal reduction of the number of granulocytes in the blood; agranulocytosis.

Granuloma—A growth or mass of granulation tissue produced in response to chronic infection, inflammation, a foreign body, or unknown causes.

Graves' disease—Disorder that causes thyrotoxicosis, goiter, and exophthalmos. Also called *exophthalmic goiter*.

Groin—The area between the abdomen and thigh.

Guillain-Barré syndrome—Nerve disease

marked by sudden numbness and weakness in the limbs that may progress to complete paralysis.

Gynecomastia—Excessive development of the breasts in the male.

Hair follicle—Sheath of tissue surrounding a hair root.

Hansen's disease—See Leprosy.

Hartnup disease—Hereditary disease in which the body has trouble processing certain chemicals, leading to mental retardation, rough skin, and problems with muscle coordination.

Healthy—Food labeling term that may be used if the food is low in fat and saturated fat and a serving does not contain more than 480 milligrams of sodium or more than 95 milligrams of cholesterol. The food must also meet requirements of 10% DV per serving of vitamin A, vitamin C, calcium, iron, protein, and fiber.

Heart attack—See Myocardial infarction.

Hematuria—Presence of blood or red blood cells in the urine.

Hemoglobin—Iron-containing substance found in red blood cells that transports oxygen from the lungs to the tissues of the body.

Hemolytic anemia—Type of anemia resulting from breakdown of red blood cells.

Hemophilia—Hereditary disease in males in which blood clotting is delayed, leading to excessive and uncontrolled bleeding even after minor injuries.

Hemorrhoids—Enlarged veins in the walls of the anus. Also called *piles*.

Hepatic—Relating to the liver.

Hepatitis—Inflammation of the liver.

Hernia, hiatal—Condition in which the stomach passes partly into the chest through the opening for the esophagus in the diaphragm.

Herpes simplex—The virus that causes "cold sores." These are an inflammation of the skin resulting in small, painful blisters. Infection may occur either in or around the mouth or, in the case of genital herpes, on the genitals (sex organs).

Herpes zoster—An infectious disease usually marked by pain and blisters along one nerve, often on the face, chest, stomach, or back. The infection is caused by the virus that also causes chickenpox. Also called *shingles*.

Heterosexual—One who is sexually attracted to persons of the opposite sex.

High blood pressure—See Hypertension.

High fiber—In food labeling, 5 grams or more of fiber per serving. (Foods making high-fiber claims must meet the definition for low fat, or the level of total fat must appear next to the high-fiber claim.)

Hirsutism—Adult male pattern of hair growth in women.

HIV (human immunodeficiency virus)—Virus that causes AIDS.

Hodgkin's disease—Malignant condition

marked by swelling of the lymph nodes, with weight loss and fever.

Homosexual—One who is sexually attracted to persons of the same sex.

Hormone—Substance produced in one part of the body (such as a gland), which then passes into the bloodstream and travels to other organs or tissues, where it carries out its effect.

Hot flashes—Sensations of heat of the face, neck, and upper body, often accompanied by sweating and flushing; commonly associated with menopause.

Hydrocortisone—See Cortisol.

Hyperactivity—Abnormally increased activity.

Hypercalcemia—Too much calcium in the blood.

Hypercalciuria—Too much calcium in the urine.

Hypercholesterolemia—Excessive amount of cholesterol in the blood.

Hyperglycemia—Abnormally high blood sugar.

Hyperkalemia—Abnormally high amount of potassium in the blood.

Hyperkeratosis—Overgrowth or thickening of the outer horny layer of the skin.

Hyperlipidemia—General term for an abnormally high level of any or all of the lipids in the blood.

Hyperphosphatemia—Too much phosphate in the blood.

Hypersensitivity—Condition in which the body has an abnormally increased reaction to a foreign substance.

Hypertension—Blood pressure in the arteries (blood vessels) that is higher than normal for the patient's age group. Hypertension may lead to a number of serious health problems. Also called *high blood pressure*.

Hyperthermia—Abnormally high body temperature.

Hyperthyroidism—Excessive secretion of thyroid hormones by the thyroid gland, causing thyrotoxicosis.

Hypocalcemia—Too little calcium in the blood.

Hypoglycemia—Abnormally low blood sugar.

Hypokalemia—Abnormally low amount of potassium in the blood.

Hypotension, orthostatic—Excessive fall in blood pressure that occurs when standing or upon standing up.

Hypothalamus—Area of the brain that controls many body functions, including body temperature, certain metabolic and endocrine processes, and some activities of the nervous system.

Hypothermia—Abnormally low body temperature.

Hypothyroidism—Condition caused by thyroid hormone deficiency, which results in a decrease in metabolism.

Hypoxia—Broad term meaning intake of oxygen or its use by the body is inadequate.

Ileostomy—Operation in which the ileum is brought through the abdominal wall to create an artificial opening. The contents of the intestine are discharged through the opening, bypassing the colon (bowel).

Ileum—Last of the three portions of the small intestine.

Immune deficiency condition—Lack of immune response to protect against infectious disease.

Immune system—Complex network of the body that defends against foreign substances or organisms that may harm the body.

Immunizing agent, active—Agent that causes the body to produce its own antibodies for protection against certain infections.

Immunocompromised—Decreased natural immunity caused by irradiation, certain medicine or diseases, or other conditions.

Immunosuppressant—Medicine that reduces the body's natural immunity.

Impair—To cause to decrease, weaken, or damage, usually because of injury or disease.

Impetigo—Contagious bacterial skin infection common in babies and children in which skin redness develops into blisters that break and form a thick crust.

Implant—1. Special form of medicine, often a small pellet or rod, that is inserted into the body or beneath the skin so that the medicine will be released continuously over a period of time. 2. To insert or graft material or an object into a body site. 3. Material or an object inserted into a body site, such as a lens implant or a breast implant. 4. Action of a fertilized ovum becoming attached to or embedded in the uterus.

Impotence—Difficulty or inability of a male to have or maintain an erection of the penis.

Incontinence—Inability to control natural passage of urine or of bowel movements.

Induce—To cause or bring about.

Infertility—Medical condition which results in the difficulty or inability of a woman to become pregnant or of a man to cause pregnancy.

Inflammation—Pain, redness, swelling, and heat in a part of the body, usually in response to injury or illness.

Inflammatory bowel disease—Irritation of the intestinal tract.

Influenza—Highly contagious respiratory virus infection, marked by coughing, headache, chills, fever, muscle pain, and general weakness. Also called *flu*.

Ingredient—One of the parts or substances that make up a mixture or compound.

Inhalation—1. Act of drawing in the breath or drawing air into the lungs. 2. Medicine that is used when breathed (inhaled) into the lungs. Some inhalations work locally in the lungs, while others produce their effects elsewhere in the body.

Inhibitor—Substance that prevents a process or reaction.

Inner ear—Inner portion of the ear; a liquid filled system of cavities and ducts that make up the organs of hearing and balance.

Insomnia—Inability to sleep or remain asleep.

Insulin—Hormone that increases the efficiency with which the body uses sugar. Injections of insulin are used in the treatment and control of diabetes mellitus (sugar diabetes).

Intra-amniotic—Within the sac that contains the fetus and amniotic fluid.

Intra-arterial—Within an artery.

Intracavernosal—Into the corpus cavernosa (cavities in the penis that, when filled with blood, produce an erection).

Intracavitary—Into a body cavity (for example, the chest cavity or bladder).

Intramuscular—Into a muscle.

Intrauterine device (IUD)—Small plastic or metal device placed in the uterus (womb) to prevent pregnancy.

Intravenous—Into a vein.

Ion—Atom or group of atoms carrying an electric charge.

Irrigation—Washing of a body cavity or wound with a stream of sterile water or a solution of a medicine.

Ischemia—Condition caused by inadequate blood flow to a part of the body; usually caused by constriction or blocking of blood vessels that supply the part of the body affected.

Jaundice—Yellowing of the eyes and skin due to excess bilirubin in the blood.

Jock itch—Ringworm of the groin.

Kala-azar—See Leishmaniasis, visceral.

Kaposi's sarcoma—Malignant tumor of blood vessels; often appears in the skin. One form occurs in immunocompromised patients, for example, transplant recipients and AIDS patients.

Keratolytic—Medicine used to soften hardened areas of the skin, such as warts.

Ketoacidosis—Type of acidosis associated with diabetes.

Lactation—Secretion of breast milk.

Larva—The immature form of life of some insects and other animal groups that hatch from eggs.

Larynx—Organ that serves as a passage for air from the pharynx to the lungs; it contains the vocal cords.

Laxative—Medicine used to encourage bowel movements.

Laxative, bulk-forming—Laxative that acts by absorbing liquid and swelling to form a soft, bulky stool. The bowel is then stimulated normally by the presence of the bulky mass.

Laxative, hyperosmotic—Laxative that acts by drawing water into the bowel from surrounding body tissues. This provides a soft stool mass and increased bowel action.

Laxative, lubricant—Laxative that acts by coating the bowel and the stool mass with a waterproof film. This keeps moisture in the stool. The stool remains soft and its passage is made easier.

Laxative, stimulant—Laxative that acts directly on the intestinal wall. The direct stimulation increases the muscle contractions that move the stool mass along. Also called *contact laxative*.

Laxative, stool softener—Laxative that acts by helping liquids mix into the stool and prevent dry, hard stool masses. The stool remains soft and its passage is made easier. Also called *emollient laxative*.

Lean—Food labeling term for seafood or game meat, meals, and main dishes. May be used if a serving contains less than 10 grams of total fat, 4.5 grams or less of saturated fat, and less than 95 milligrams of cholesterol. Seafood and game meat must meet these criteria per 100 grams of food. Meals and main dishes must meet these criteria per 100 grams of food and per labeled serving.

Legionnaires' disease—Lung infection caused by a certain bacterium.

Leishmaniasis, visceral—Tropical disease, transmitted by sandfly bites, which causes liver and spleen enlargement, anemia, weight loss, and fever. Also called *black fever*, *Dumdum fever*, or *kala-azar*.

Lennox-Gastaut syndrome—Type of childhood epilepsy.

Leprosy—Chronic infectious disease characterized by lesions, especially in the skin and nerves, leading to loss of feeling, paralysis in the hands and feet, and deformity. Also called *Hansen's disease.*

Less cholesterol—In food labeling, at least 25 percent less cholesterol and 2 grams or less of saturated fat per serving than the reference food.

Less fat—In food labeling, at least 25 percent less fat per serving than the reference food.

Less saturated fat—In food labeling, at least 25 percent less fat per serving than the reference food.

Less sodium—In food labeling, at least 25 percent less sodium per serving than the reference food.

Less sugar—In food labeling, at least 25 percent less sugar per serving than the reference food.

Leukemia—Disease of the blood and bone marrow in which too many white blood cells are produced, resulting in anemia, bleeding, and low resistance to infections.

Leukocyte—White blood cell.

Leukoderma—See Vitiligo.

Leukopenia—Abnormal reduction in the total number of leukocytes in the blood.

Lipid—Term applied generally to dietary fat or fatlike substances not soluble in water.

Local effect—Affecting only the area to which something is being applied.

Low calorie—In food labeling, 40 calories or

less per serving. However, for small servings (30 grams or less or 2 tablespoons or less), low calorie is 40 calories or less per 50 grams of the food.

Low cholesterol—In food labeling, 20 milligrams or less of cholesterol and 2 grams or less of saturated fat per serving. However, for small servings (30 grams or less or 2 tablespoons or less), low cholesterol is 20 milligrams or less of cholesterol per 50 grams of the food and 2 grams or less of saturated fat per serving.

Low fat—In food labeling, 3 grams or less of fat per serving. However, for small servings (30 grams or less or 2 tablespoons or less), low fat is 3 grams or less of fat per 50 grams of the food.

Low saturated fat—One gram or less of fat per serving and not more than 15 percent of calories from saturated fatty acids.

Low sodium—In food labeling, 140 milligrams or less of sodium per serving. However, for small servings (30 grams or less or 2 tablespoons or less), low sodium is 140 milligrams or less of sodium per 50 grams of the food.

Lugol's solution—Transparent, deep brown liquid containing iodine and potassium iodide.

Lupus—See Lupus erythematosus, systemic.

Lupus erythematosus, systemic—Chronic inflammatory disease most often affecting the skin, joints, and various internal organs.

Also called *lupus* or *SLE* (systemic lupus erythematosus).

Lymph—Fluid that bathes the tissues. It is formed in tissue spaces in all parts of the body and circulated by the lymphatic system.

Lymphatic system—Network of vessels that conveys lymph from the spaces between the cells of the body back to the bloodstream.

Lymph node—A small rounded body found at intervals along the lymphatic system. The nodes act as filters for the lymph by keeping bacteria and other foreign particles from entering the bloodstream. They also produce lymphocytes.

Lymphocyte—Any of a number of white blood cells found in the blood, lymph, and lymphatic tissues. They are involved in immunity.

Lymphoma—Malignant tumor of lymph nodes or tissue.

Lyse—To cause breakdown. In cells, damage or rupture of the membrane results in destruction of the cell.

Macrobiotic—Vegetarian diet consisting mostly of whole grains.

Malaria—Tropical blood infection caused by a protozoa; symptoms include chills, fever, sweats, headaches, and anemia. Malaria is spread to humans by the bite of an infected mosquito.

Malignant—Describing a condition that becomes continually worse if untreated; also used to mean cancerous.

Malnutrition—Condition caused by unbalanced or insufficient diet.

Mammogram—X-ray picture of the breast.

Mania—Mental state in which fast talking and excited feelings or actions are out of control.

Mast cells—Cells in the connective tissue that store histamine; they release substances that bring about inflammation and produce signs of allergic reactions.

Mastocytosis—Accumulation of too many mast cells in tissues.

Mediate—To bring about or accomplish indirectly.

Megavitamin therapy—Taking very large doses of vitamins to prevent or treat certain medical problems.

Melanoma—Highly malignant cancer tumor, usually occurring on the skin.

Meniérè's disease—Disease affecting the inner ear that is characterized by ringing in the ears, hearing loss, and dizziness.

Meningitis—Inflammation of the tissues that surround the brain and spinal cord.

Menopause—The time in a woman's life when the ovaries no longer produce an egg cell at regular times and menstruation stops.

Methemoglobin—Substance formed when hemoglobin has been oxidized; in this form, hemoglobin cannot act as an oxygen carrier.

Methemoglobinemia—Presence of methemoglobin in the blood.

Middle ear—Chamber of the ear lying behind the eardrum and containing the structures that conduct sound.

Migraine—Throbbing headache, usually affecting one side of the head; often accompanied by nausea, vomiting, and sensitivity to light.

Mineral—One of many elements needed in small amounts for many body functions, including blood clotting, muscle movement, and fluid balance.

Miotic—Medicine used in the eye that causes the pupil to constrict (become smaller).

Mongolism—See Down syndrome.

Mono—See Mononucleosis.

Monoclonal—Derived from a single cell; related to production of drugs by genetic engineering, such as monoclonal antibodies.

Mononucleosis—Infectious viral disease occurring mostly in adolescents and young adults, marked by fever, sore throat, swelling of the lymph nodes in the neck and armpits, and by severe fatigue. Also called *mono* or *glandular fever*.

More fiber—See Added fiber.

Motility—Ability to move without outside aid, force, or cause.

Motor—Relating to structures that bring about movement, such as nerves and muscles.

Mucolytic—Medicine that breaks down or dissolves mucus.

Mucosal—Relating to the mucous membrane.

Mucous membrane—Moist layer of tissue surrounding or lining many body structures and cavities, including the mouth, lips, inside of nose, anus, and vagina.

Mucus—Thick fluid produced by the mucous membranes and glands.

Multiple sclerosis (MS)—Chronic, inflammatory nerve disease marked by weakness, unsteadiness, shakiness, and speech and vision problems.

Myasthenia gravis—Chronic disease marked by abnormal weakness, and sometimes paralysis, of certain muscles.

Mydriatic—Medicine used in the eye that causes the pupil to dilate (become larger).

Myelogram—X-ray picture of the spinal cord.

Myeloma, multiple—Cancerous bone marrow disease.

Myocardial infarction—Interruption of blood supply to the heart, leading to sudden, severe chest pain, and damage to the heart muscle. Also called *heart attack*.

Myocardial reinfarction prophylactic—Medicine used to help prevent additional heart attacks in patients who have already had one attack.

Myotonia congenita—Hereditary muscle disorder marked by difficulty in relaxing a muscle or releasing a grip after any strong effort.

Narcolepsy—Extreme tendency to fall asleep suddenly.

Nasal—Relating to the nose.

Nasogastric (NG) tube—Tube that is inserted through the nose, down the throat, and into the stomach. It may be used to remove fluid or gas from the stomach or to administer medicine, food, fluid, or nutrients to the patient.

Nebulizer—Instrument that administers liquid in the form of a fine spray.

Necrosis—Death of tissue, cells, or a part of a structure or organ, surrounded by healthy parts.

Neoplasm—New and abnormal growth of tissue in or on a part of the body, in which the multiplication of cells is uncontrolled and progressive. Also called *tumor*.

Nephron—Unit of the kidney that acts as a filter of the blood in forming urine.

Neuralgia—Severe stabbing or throbbing pain along the course of one or more nerves.

Neuralgia, trigeminal—Severe burning or stabbing pain along certain nerves in the face. Also called *tic douloureux*.

Neural tube defects—Severe, abnormal conditions resulting when the nerve tract in the fetus fails to close fully. See Spina bifida.

Neuritis, optic—Disease of the nerves in the eye.

Neuritis, peripheral—Inflammation of terminal nerves or the nerve endings, usually associated with pain, muscle wasting, and loss of reflexes.

Neutropenia—Abnormally small number of neutrophils in the blood.

Neutrophil—The most common type of granulocyte; important in the body's protection against infection.

No added sugar—In food labeling, no sugars added to food during processing or packing. This includes ingredients that contain sugars—for example, fruit juices, applesauce, or dried fruit.

Nodule—Small, rounded mass, lump, or swelling.

Nonsuppurative—Not discharging pus.

No sugar added—See No added sugar.

NSAID (nonsteroidal anti-inflammatory drug)—See Anti-inflammatory, nonsteroidal.

Nucleus—The part of the cell that contains the chromosomes.

Nutrition Labeling and Education Act (NLEA) of 1990—The law that required the Food and Drug Administration to develop new labeling requirements for foods and dietary supplements.

Nystagmus—Rapid, rhythmic, involuntary movements of the eyeball; may be from side to side, up and down, or around.

Obesity—Excess accumulation of fat in the body along with an increase in body weight that exceeds the healthy range for the body's frame.

Obstetrics—Field of medicine concerned with

the care of women during pregnancy and childbirth.

Obstruction—Something that blocks or closes up a passage or structure.

Occlusive dressing—Dressing (such as plastic kitchen wrap) that completely cuts off air to the skin.

Occult—Concealed, hidden, or of unknown cause; cannot be seen by the human eye; detectable only by microscope or chemical testing, as for occult blood in the stools or feces.

Ophthalmic—Relating to the eye.

Opioid—1. Any synthetic narcotic with opium-like actions; not derived from opium. 2. Natural chemicals that produce opium-like effects by acting at the same cell sites where opium exerts action.

Oral—Relating to the mouth.

Orchitis—Inflammation of the testis.

Organic—1. In nutrition, a term used to describe plants that have been treated with animal or vegetable fertilizers instead of chemicals. 2. In chemistry, refers to substances that contain carbon.

Osteitis deformans—See Paget's disease.

Osteomalacia—Softening of the bones due to lack of vitamin D.

Osteoporosis—Loss of calcium from bone tissue, resulting in bones that are brittle and easily fractured.

OTC (over the counter)—Refers to medicine or devices available without a prescription.

Otic—Relating to the ear.

Otitis media—Inflammation of the middle ear.

Ototoxicity—Having a harmful effect on the organs or nerves of the ear concerned with hearing and balance.

Ovary—Female sex organ that produces egg cells and sex hormones. The two ovaries are in the lower abdomen, one on each side.

Overactive thyroid—See Hyperthyroidism.

Ovulation—Process by which an ovum is released from the ovary. In human menstruating females, this usually occurs once a month.

Ovum—Mature female sex or reproductive cell, or egg cell. It is capable of developing into a new organism if fertilized.

Paget's disease—Chronic bone disease, marked by thickening of the bones and severe pain. Also called *osteitis deformans*.

Pancreatitis—Inflammation of the pancreas.

Pancytopenia—Reduction in the number of red cells, all types of white cells, and platelets in the blood.

Paralysis agitans—See Parkinson's disease.

Parathyroid glands—Four small bodies situated beside the thyroid gland; secrete parathyroid hormone that regulates calcium and phosphorus metabolism.

Parenteral—Any method of administering medicine when the medicine cannot be given by mouth; most often refers to injecting a medicine into the body using a needle and syringe.

Parkinsonism—See Parkinson's disease.

Parkinson's disease—Brain disease marked by tremor (shaking), stiffness, and difficulty in moving. Also called *Parkinsonism, paralysis agitans,* or *shaking palsy.*

Patent ductus arteriosus (PDA)—Condition in babies in which an important blood vessel adjacent to the heart fails to close as it should, resulting in faulty circulation and serious health problems.

Pediculicide—Medicine that kills lice.

Pediculosis—Infestation of the body, pubis, or scalp with lice.

Pellagra—Disease caused by too little niacin, which results in scaly skin, diarrhea, and mental depression.

Pemphigus—Skin disease marked by successive outbreaks of blisters.

Peptic ulcer—Open sore in esophagus, stomach, or duodenum.

Peritoneum—Membrane sac lining the abdominal wall and covering the liver, stomach, spleen, gallbladder, and intestines.

Peritonitis—Inflammation of the peritoneum.

Peyronie's disease—Dense, fiber-like growth in the penis, which can be felt as an irregular hard lump, and which usually causes bending and pain when the penis is erect.

Pharynx—Space just behind the mouth that serves as a passageway for food from the mouth to the esophagus and for air from the nose and mouth to the larynx.

Phenol—Substance used as a preservative for some injectable medicines.

Pheochromocytoma—Tumor of the adrenal medulla.

Phlebitis—Inflammation of a vein.

Phlegm—Thick mucus produced in the respiratory passages.

Piles—See Hemorrhoids.

Pituitary gland—Pea-sized body located at the base of the skull. It produces a number of hormones that are essential to normal body growth and functioning.

Placebo—Medicine that, unknown to the patient, has no active medicinal substance; its use may relieve or improve a condition because the patient believes it will. Also called *sugar pill*.

Plaque, dental—Mixture of saliva, bacteria, and carbohydrates that forms on the teeth, leading to caries (cavities) and gum disease.

Platelet—Small, disk-shaped body found in the blood that plays an important role in blood clotting.

Platelet aggregation inhibitor—Medicine used to help prevent the platelets in the blood from clumping together. This effect reduces the chance of heart attack or stroke in certain patients.

Pleura—Membrane covering the lungs and lining the chest cavity.

Pneumococcal—Relating to certain bacteria that cause pneumonia.

Pneumocystis carinii—Organism that causes pneumocystis carinii pneumonia.

Pneumocystis carinii pneumonia—A pulmonary disease of infants and weakened persons, including those with AIDS or those receiving drugs that weaken the immune system.

Polymorphous light eruption—A skin problem in certain people, which results from exposure to sunlight.

Polymyalgia rheumatica—A rheumatic disease, most common in elderly patients, which causes aching and stiffness in the shoulders and hips.

Polyp—Tumor or mass of tissue attached with a stalk or broad base; found in cavities such as the nose, uterus, or rectum.

Porphyria—A group of uncommon, usually inherited diseases of defective porphyrin metabolism.

Porphyrin—One of a number of pigments occurring in living organisms throughout nature; porphyrins are constituents of bile pigment, hemoglobin, and certain enzymes.

Potency—Strength of a medicine, chemical, or vitamin that will bring about a certain effect.

Prevent—To stop or to keep from happening.

Priapism—Prolonged abnormal, painful erection of the penis.

Proctitis—Inflammation of the rectum.

Progesterone—Natural steroid hormone responsible for preparing the uterus for pregnancy. If fertilization occurs, progesterone's actions carry on or maintain the pregnancy.

Progestin—A natural or synthetic hormone that has progesterone-like actions.

Prolactin—Hormone secreted by the pituitary gland that stimulates and maintains milk flow in women following childbirth.

Prolactinoma—A pituitary tumor; results in secretion of excess prolactin.

Prophylactic—1. Agent or medicine used to prevent the occurrence of a specific condition. 2. Condom.

Prostate—Gland surrounding the neck of the male urethra just below the base of the bladder. It secretes a fluid that constitutes a major portion of the semen.

Prosthesis—Any artificial substitute for a missing body part.

Protein—One of a class of compounds that contain carbon, hydrogen, nitrogen, oxygen, and sometimes other elements. Proteins make up the greatest part of plant and animal tissue. They are a source of energy for animals and humans.

Protozoa—Tiny, one-celled animals; some cause diseases in humans.

Psoralen—Chemical found in plants and used in certain perfumes and medicines. Exposure to a psoralen and then to sunlight may increase the risk of severe burning.

Psoriasis—Chronic skin disease marked by itchy, scaly, red patches.

Psychosis—Severe mental illness marked by loss of contact with reality, often involving delusions, hallucinations, and disordered thinking.

Purity—Free from contamination.

Purpura—Condition marked by bleeding into the skin; skin rash or spots are first red, darken to purple, then fade to brownish-yellow.

PUVA—Treatment for psoriasis by use of a psoralen, such as methoxsalen or trioxsalen, and long-wave ultraviolet light.

Rachischisis—See Spina bifida.

Radiopaque agent—Substance that makes it easier to see an area of the body with x-rays. Radiopaque agents are used to help diagnose a variety of medical problems.

Radiopharmaceutical—Radioactive agent used to diagnose certain medical problems or treat certain diseases.

Raynaud's syndrome—Condition marked by paleness, numbness, and discomfort in the fingers when they are exposed to cold.

Recommended Dietary Allowances (RDAs)—In the U.S., the amount of vitamins and minerals needed to provide for adequate nutrition in most healthy persons. RDAs for a given nutrient may vary depending on a person's age, sex, and physical condition (for example, pregnancy).

Recommended Nutrient Intakes (RNIs)—In

Canada, values used to determine the amounts of vitamins, minerals, and protein needed to provide adequate nutrition and lessen the risk of chronic disease.

Rectal—Relating to the rectum.

Reduced calories—See Fewer calories.

Reduced cholesterol—See Less cholesterol.

Reduced fat—See Less fat.

Reduced saturated fat—See Less saturated fat.

Reduced sodium—See Less sodium.

Reduced sugar—See Less sugar.

Reference food—A basic food item. In food labeling, a reference food is compared against the same food that has had something added to it or taken away from it.

Renal—Relating to the kidneys.

Reye's syndrome—Serious disease affecting the liver and brain that sometimes occurs after a virus infection, such as influenza or chickenpox. It occurs most often in young children and teenagers. The first sign of Reye's syndrome is usually severe, prolonged vomiting.

Rheumatic heart disease—Heart disease marked by scarring and chronic inflammation of the heart and its valves, occurring after rheumatic fever.

Rhinitis—Inflammation of the mucous membrane inside the nose.

Rickets—Bone disease usually caused by too little vitamin D, resulting in soft and malformed bones.

Ringworm—See Tinea.

Risk—The possibility of injury or of suffering harm.

River blindness—Tropical disease produced by infection with worms of the Onchocerca type. The condition usually causes severe itching and may cause blindness. Also called *Roble's disease, blinding filarial disease,* and *craw-craw.*

Rosacea—Skin disease of the face, usually in middle-aged and older persons. Also called *adult acne.*

Sarcoidosis—Chronic disorder in which the lymph nodes in many parts of the body are enlarged, and small fleshy swellings develop in the lungs, liver, and spleen.

Saturated fat—In chemistry, a fat that has all of the possible hydrogen atoms present on the carbon atoms and no double or triple bonds between the carbon atoms.

Saturated fat free—In food labeling, less than 0.5 grams of fat and less than 0.5 grams trans fatty acid per serving.

Scabicide—Medicine used to treat scabies (itch mite) infection.

Scabies—Contagious dermatitis caused by a mite burrowing into the skin; characterized by tiny skin eruptions and severe itching.

Schistosomiasis—Tropical infection in which worms enter the skin from infested water and settle in the bladder or intestines, causing inflammation and scarring. Also called *bilharziasis.*

Schizophrenia—Severe mental disorder in which thinking, mood, and behavior are disturbed.

Scintigram—Image obtained by detecting radiation emitted from a radiopharmaceutical introduced into the body.

Scleroderma—Chronic disease first characterized by hardening, thickening, and shrinking of the skin; later, certain organs also are affected.

Scotoma—Area of decreased vision or total loss of vision in a part of the visual field; blind spot.

Scrotum—Sac that holds the testes (male sex glands).

Scurvy—Disease caused by a deficiency of vitamin C (ascorbic acid), marked by bleeding gums, bleeding beneath the skin, and body weakness.

Sebaceous gland—Skin gland that secretes sebum.

Seborrhea—Skin condition caused by the excess release of sebum from the sebaceous glands, accompanied by dandruff and oily skin.

Sebum—Fatty secretion produced by sebaceous (oil) glands of the skin.

Secretion—1. Process in which a gland in the body or on the surface of the body releases a substance for use. 2. The substance released by the gland.

Sedative-hypnotic—Medicine used to treat

excessive nervousness, restlessness, or insomnia.

Sedation—A profoundly relaxed or calmed state.

Seizure—A sudden attack or convulsion, as in epilepsy or other disorders.

Semen—Fluid released from the penis at sexual climax. It is made up of sperm suspended in secretions from the reproductive tract.

Severe—Of a great degree, such as very serious pain or distress.

Shaking palsy—See Parkinson's disease.

Shingles—See Herpes zoster.

Shock—Severe disruption of cellular metabolism associated with reduced blood volume and blood pressure too low to supply adequate blood to the tissues.

Shunt—Surgical tube used to transfer blood or other fluid from one part of the body to another.

SIADH (secretion of inappropriate antidiuretic hormone) syndrome—Disease in which the body retains (keeps) more fluid than normal.

Sickle cell anemia—Hereditary disorder that predominantly affects blacks; caused by abnormal hemoglobin. The name comes from the sickle-shaped red blood cells found in the blood of patients.

Sinusitis—Inflammation of a sinus.

Sjögren's syndrome—Condition usually occurring in older women, marked by dry eyes, dry mouth, and rheumatoid arthritis.

Skeletal muscle relaxant—Medicine used to relax certain muscles and help relieve the pain and discomfort caused by strains, sprains, or other injury to the muscles.

SLE—See Lupus erythematosus, systemic.

Sodium free—In food labeling, less than 5 milligrams of sodium per serving.

Soluble—Able to be dissolved in a fluid.

Spasticity—Increase in normal muscular tone, causing stiff, awkward movements.

Spastic paralysis—Paralysis marked by muscle rigidity or spasticity in the part of the body that is paralyzed.

Sperm—Mature male reproductive or sex cell.

Spermicide—Substance that kills sperm.

Spina bifida—Birth defect in which the infant's spinal cord is partially exposed through a hole in the backbone. Also called *rachischisis.*

Stenosis—Abnormal narrowing of a passage or duct of the body.

Sterility—1. Inability to produce offspring. 2. The state of being free of living microorganisms.

Stimulant, respiratory—Medicine used to stimulate breathing.

Stomatitis—Inflammation of the mucous membrane of the mouth.

Strength—In nutrition, the measure of a vitamin's health value.

Streptokinase—Enzyme that dissolves blood clots.

Stroke—Very serious event which occurs when an artery to the brain becomes clogged by a blood clot or bursts and causes hemorrhage. Stroke can affect speech, memory, behavior, and other life patterns, and may result in paralysis. Also called *apoplexy*.

Stye—Infection of one or more sebaceous glands of the eyelid, marked by swelling.

Subcutaneous—Under the skin.

Sublingual—Under the tongue. A sublingual medicine is taken by placing it under the tongue and letting it slowly dissolve.

Sudden infant death syndrome (SIDS)—Death of an infant, usually while asleep, from an unknown cause. Also called *crib death* or *cot death*.

Sugar diabetes—See Diabetes mellitus.

Sugar free—In food labeling, less than 0.5 grams of sugar per serving.

Sugar pill—See Placebo.

Sulfite—Type of preservative; causes allergic reactions, such as asthma, in sensitive patients.

Sunscreen—Substance, usually a cream or lotion, that blocks ultraviolet light and helps prevent sunburn when applied to the skin.

Suppository—Mass of medicated material shaped for insertion into the rectum, vagina, or urethra. Suppository is solid at room temperature but melts at body temperature.

Suppressant—Medicine that stops an action or condition.

Suspension—A form of medicine in which the drug is mixed with a liquid but is not dissolved in it. When left standing, particles settle at the bottom of the liquid and the top portion turns clear. When shaken it is ready for use.

Syncope—Sudden loss of consciousness due to inadequate blood flow to the brain; fainting.

Syphilis—An infectious disease, usually transmitted by sexual contact. The three stages of the disease may be separated by months or years.

Syringe—Device used to inject liquids into the body, remove material from a part of the body, or wash out a body cavity.

Systemic—For general effects throughout the body; applies to most medicines when taken by mouth or given by injection.

Tachycardia—Abnormal rapid beating of the heart, usually at a rate over 100 beats per minute in adults.

Temporomandibular joint (TMJ)—Hinge that connects the lower jaw to the skull.

Tendinitis—Inflammation of a tendon.

Teratogenic—Causing abnormal development in an embryo or fetus, resulting in birth defects.

Testosterone—Principal male sex hormone.

Tetany—Condition marked by spasm and twitching of the muscles, particularly those of the hands, feet, and face; caused by a decrease in the calcium ion concentration in the blood.

Therapeutic—Relating to the treatment of a specific condition.

Thimerosal—Chemical used as a preservative in some medicines, and as an antiseptic and disinfectant.

Thrombolytic agent—Substance that dissolves blood clots.

Thrombophlebitis—Inflammation of a vein accompanied by the formation of a blood clot.

Thrombus—Blood clot that obstructs a blood vessel or a cavity of the heart.

Thrush—See Candidiasis of the mouth.

Thyroid gland—Gland in the lower front of the neck. It releases thyroid hormones, which control body metabolism.

Thyrotoxicosis—Condition resulting from excessive amounts of thyroid hormones in the blood, causing increased metabolism, fast heartbeat, tremors, nervousness, and increased sweating.

Tic—Repeated involuntary movement or spasm of a muscle.

Tic douloureux—See Neuralgia, trigeminal.

Tinea—Fungus infection of the surface of the skin, particularly the scalp, feet, and nails. Also called *ringworm*.

Tone—The slight, continuous tension present in resting muscles.

Topical—For local effects when applied directly to the skin.

Tourette's disorder—Condition usually marked with motor tics (jerking movements) and vocal tics (grunts, sniffs). Also called *Gilles de la Tourette syndrome.*

Toxemia—Blood poisoning caused by bacterial production of toxins.

Toxemia of pregnancy—Condition occurring in pregnant women marked by hypertension, edema, excess protein in the urine, convulsions, and possibly coma.

Toxic—Poisonous; related to or caused by a toxin or poison.

Toxin—A substance produced by an animal or plant that is poisonous to another organism.

Toxoplasmosis—Disease caused by a blood protozoan, usually transmitted to humans from cats or by eating raw meat; generally the symptoms are mild and self-limited.

Tracheostomy—A surgical opening through the throat into the trachea (windpipe) to bypass an obstruction to breathing.

Tranquilizer—Medicine that produces a calming effect. It is used to relieve mental anxiety and tension.

Transdermal—A means of administering medicine into the body by use of skin patches or disks, or ointment; medicine contained in the patch or disk or the ointment is absorbed through the skin.

Trichomoniasis—Infection of the vagina resulting in inflammation of genital tissues and discharge. It can be passed on to males.

Triglyceride—A molecular form in which fats are present in food and the body; triglycerides are stored in the body as fat.

Trypanosome fever—See Trypanosomiasis, African.

Trypanosomiasis, African—Tropical disease, transmitted by tsetse fly bites, which causes fever, headache, and chills, followed by enlarged lymph nodes and anemia. Months or even years later, the disease affects the central nervous system, causing drowsiness and lethargy, coma, and death. Also called *African sleeping sickness.*

Tuberculosis (TB)—Infectious disease which may affect any organ but most commonly the lungs; symptoms include fever, night sweats, weight loss, and spitting up blood.

Tumor—Abnormal growth or enlargement in or on a part of the body.

Tyramine—Chemical present in many foods and beverages. Its structure and action in the body are similar to epinephrine.

Ulcer—Open sore or break in the skin or mucous membrane; often fails to heal and is accompanied by inflammation.

Ulcerative colitis—Chronic, recurrent inflammation and ulceration of the colon.

Ulceration—1. Formation or development of

an ulcer. 2. Condition of an area marked with ulcers loosely associated with one another.

Underactive thyroid—See Hypothyroidism.

Ureter—Tube through which urine passes from the kidney to the bladder.

Urethra—Tube through which urine passes from the bladder to the outside of the body.

Urticaria—Hives; an eruption of itching wheals on the skin.

USRDA—Labeling term formerly used to indicate how much of a nutrient a serving provided. This term is now stated as Daily Value (DV).

Vaccine—Medicine given by mouth or by injection to produce immunity to a certain infection.

Vaccinia—The skin and sometimes body reactions associated with smallpox vaccine. Also called *cowpox*.

Vaginal—Relating to the vagina.

Varicella—Very infectious viral disease marked by fever and itchy rash that develops into blisters and then scabs. Also called *chickenpox*.

Vascular—Relating to the blood vessels.

Vasodilator—Medicine that dilates the blood vessels, permitting increased blood flow.

Ventricular fibrillation—Life-threatening condition of fine, quivering, irregular movements of many individual muscle fibers of the ventricular muscle; replaces the normal heartbeat and interrupts pumping function.

Ventricle—A small cavity, such as one of the two lower chambers of the heart or one of the several cavities of the brain.

Vertigo—Sensation of whirling motion or dizziness, either of oneself or of one's surroundings.

Very low sodium—In food labeling, 35 milligrams or less of sodium per serving. However, for small servings (30 grams or less or 2 tablespoons or less), very low sodium is 35 milligrams or less of sodium per 50 grams of the food.

Veterinary—Relating to animals and their diseases and treatment.

Virus—Any of a group of simple microbes too small to be seen by a light microscope. They can grow and reproduce only in living cells. Many cause diseases in humans, including the common cold.

Vitamin—Any of a group of substances, needed in small amounts only, for growth and health. Vitamins are usually found naturally in food, but may also be man-made.

Vitamin, natural—A vitamin that comes from natural sources such as plants.

Vitamin, synthetic—A vitamin that does not come from natural sources, but instead is man-made.

Vitamins, fat-soluble—Vitamins that can be dissolved in fat (vitamins A, D, E, K). They are stored in fat tissue.

Vitamins, water-soluble—Vitamins that can be dissolved in water (vitamin C and the

B-complex vitamins). They are stored in small amounts by the body.

Vitiligo—Condition in which some areas of skin lose pigment and turn white. Also called *leukoderma.*

von Willebrand's disease—Hereditary blood disease in which blood clotting is delayed, leading to excessive and uncontrolled bleeding even after minor injuries.

Water diabetes—See Diabetes insipidus.

Water pill—See Diuretic.

Wheal—Temporary, small, raised area of the skin, usually accompanied by itching or burning; welt.

Wheezing—A whistling sound made when there is difficulty in breathing.

White mouth—See Candidiasis of the mouth.

Wilson's disease—Inborn defect in the body's ability to process copper. Too much copper may lead to jaundice, cirrhosis, mental retardation, or symptoms like those of Parkinson's disease.

Without added sugar—See No added sugar.

Zollinger-Ellison syndrome—Disorder in which the stomach produces too much acid, leading to ulcers.

CONTRIBUTORS

USP People 1990–1995

OFFICERS

Mark Novitch, M.D., *President*, Washington, DC

Donald R. Bennett, M.D., Ph.D., *Vice-President*, Chicago, IL

John T. Fay, Jr., Ph.D., *Treasurer*, San Clemente, CA

Arthur Hull Hayes, Jr., M.D., *Past President*, New Rochelle, NY

Jerome A. Halperin, *Secretary*, Rockville, MD

BOARD OF TRUSTEES

James T. Doluisio, Ph.D.[1], *Chair*, Austin, TX

Donald R. Bennett, M.D., Ph.D., *ex officio*, Chicago, IL

John V. Bergen, Ph.D.[2], *Vice Chair*, Villanova, PA

Edwin D. Bransome, Jr., M.D.[3], Augusta, GA

Jordan L. Cohen, Ph.D.[1], Lexington, KY

J. Richard Crout, M.D.[3], Rockville, MD

John T. Fay, Jr., Ph.D., *ex officio*, San Clemente, CA

Arthur Hull Hayes, Jr., M.D., *ex officio*, New Rochelle, NY

Joseph A. Mollica, Ph.D.[2], Wilmington, DE

Grace Powers Monaco, J.D.[4], Washington, DC

Mark Novitch, M.D., *ex officio*, Washington, DC

[1]Representing pharmacy.
[2]At large.
[3]Representing medicine.
[4]Public member.

GENERAL COMMITTEE OF REVISION

---

[5]12601 Twinbrook Parkway, Rockville, MD 20852.
[6]Deceased.

Leon Ellenbogen, Ph.D., Clifton, NJ
R. Michael Enzinger, Ph.D., (1990–1992), Kalamazoo, MI
Clyde R. Erskine, B.S., M.B.A., Newtown Square, PA
Edward A. Fitzgerald, Ph.D., Bethesda, MD
Everett Flanigan, Ph.D., Kankakee, IL
Klaus G. Florey, Ph.D., Princeton, NJ
Thomas S. Foster, Pharm.D., Lexington, KY
Joseph F. Gallelli, Ph.D., Bethesda, MD
Robert L. Garnick, Ph.D., So. San Francisco, CA
Douglas D. Glover, M.D., R.Ph., Morgantown, WV
Alan M. Goldberg, Ph.D., Baltimore, MD
Burton J. Goldstein, M.D., Williams Island, FL
Dennis K. J. Gorecki, Ph.D., Saskatoon, Saskatchewan, Canada
Michael J. Groves, Ph.D., Lake Forest, IL
Robert M. Guthrie, M.D., Columbus, OH
Samir A. Hanna, Ph.D., Lawrenceville, NJ
Stanley L. Hem, Ph.D., West Lafayette, IN
Joy Hochstadt, Ph.D., New York, NY
David W. Hughes, Ph.D., (1990–1993), Nepean, Ontario, Canada
Norman C. Jamieson, Ph.D., St. Louis, MO
Richard D. Johnson, Pharm.D., Ph.D., Kansas City, MO
Judith K. Jones, M.D., Ph.D., Arlington, VA
Stanley A. Kaplan, Ph.D., Baltimore, MD
Herbert E. Kaufman, M.D., New Orleans, LA
Donald Kaye, M.D., Philadelphia, PA
Paul E. Kennedy, Ph.D., West Conshohocken, PA
Jay S. Keystone, M.D., Toronto, Ontario, Canada
Rosalyn C. King, Pharm.D., M.P.H., Silver Spring, MD
Gordon L. Klein, M.D., Galveston, TX
Joseph E. Knapp, Ph.D., Pittsburgh, PA

John B. Landis, Ph.D., (1990–1992), Kalamazoo, MI
Thomas P. Layloff, Ph.D., St. Louis, MO
Lewis J. Leeson, Ph.D., Summit, NJ
John W. Levchuk, Ph.D., Rockville, MD
Robert D. Lindeman, M.D., Albuquerque, NM
Charles H. Lochmüller, Ph.D., Durham, NC
Edward G. Lovering, Ph.D., Nepean, Ontario,
   Canada
Catherine M. MacLeod, M.D., Chicago, IL
Carol S. Marcus, Ph.D., M.D., Torrance, CA
Tibor I. Matula, Ph.D., (1993–), Ottawa, Ontario,
   Canada
Thomas Medwick, Ph.D., Piscataway, NJ
Robert F. Morrissey, Ph.D., New Brunswick, NJ
Terry E. Munson, B.S., Fairfax, VA
Harold S. Nelson, M.D., Denver, CO
Wendel L. Nelson, Ph.D., Seattle, WA
Maria I. New, M.D., New York, NY
Sharon C. Northup, Ph.D., Round Lake, IL
Jeffery L. Otto, Ph.D., (1992–), Broomfield, CO
Garnet E. Peck, Ph.D., West Lafayette, IN
Robert V. Petersen, Ph.D., Salt Lake City, UT
Rosemary C. Polomano, R.N., M.S.N.,
   Philadelphia, PA
Thomas P. Reinders, Pharm.D., Richmond, VA
Christopher T. Rhodes, Ph.D., West Kingston, RI
Joseph R. Robinson, Ph.D., Madison, WI
Lary A. Robinson, M.D., Tampa, FL
David B. Roll, Ph.D., Salt Lake City, UT
Theodore J. Roseman, Ph.D., Round Lake, IL
Sanford H. Roth, M.D., Phoenix, AZ
Leonard P. Rybak, M.D., Springfield, IL
Ronald J. Sawchuk, Ph.D., Minneapolis, MN
Gordon D. Schiff, M.D., Chicago, IL
Andrew J. Schmitz, Jr., M.S.[6], (1990–1992),
   Huntington, NY

---

[6]Deceased.

EXECUTIVE COMMITTEE OF REVISION (1994–1995)

Jerome A. Halperin, *Chair*

Norman W. Atwater, Ph.D.
Clyde R. Erskine, B.S., M.B.A.
Burton J. Goldstein, M.D.
Robert V. Petersen, Ph.D.
Robert S. Stern, M.D.
Paul F. White, Ph.D., M.D.

DRUG INFORMATION DIVISION EXECUTIVE COMMITTEE (1994–1995)

Herbert S. Carlin, D.Sc., *Chair*

James C. Boylan, Ph.D.
Sebastian G. Ciancio, D.D.S.
Lloyd E. Davis, D.V.M., Ph.D.
Jay S. Keystone, M.D.
Robert D. Lindeman, M.D.
Maria I. New, M.D.
Rosemary C. Polomano, R.N., M.S.N.
Thomas P. Reinders, Pharm.D.
Gordon D. Schiff, M.D.
Albert L. Sheffer, M.D.
Theodore G. Tong, Pharm.D.
Robert E. Vestal, M.D.
John W. Yarbro, M.D., Ph.D.

DRUG STANDARDS DIVISION EXECUTIVE COMMITTEE (1994–1995)

James T. Stewart, Ph.D., *Chair*

Jerry R. Allison, Ph.D.
Judy P. Boehlert, Ph.D.
Capt. William H. Briner, B.S.
Herbert S. Carlin, D.Sc.
Lester Chafetz, Ph.D.

Zak T. Chowhan, Ph.D.
Murray S. Cooper, Ph.D.
Klaus G. Florey, Ph.D.
Joseph F. Gallelli, Ph.D.
Robert L. Garnick, Ph.D.
Thomas P. Layloff, Ph.D.
Lewis J. Leeson, Ph.D.
Thomas Medwick, Ph.D.
Robert F. Morrissey, Ph.D.
Sharon C. Northup, Ph.D.
Ralph F. Shangraw, Ph.D.

DRUG NOMENCLATURE COMMITTEE (1994–1995)

Herbert S. Carlin, D.Sc., *Chair*

William M. Heller, Ph.D., *Consultant/Advisor*

Lester Chafetz, Ph.D.
Lloyd E. Davis, D.V.M., Ph.D.
Everett Flanigan, Ph.D.
Douglas D. Glover, M.D.
Richard D. Johnson, Pharm.D., Ph.D.
Edward G. Lovering, Ph.D.
Rosemary C. Polomano, R.N., M.S.N.
Thomas P. Reinders, Pharm.D.
Eric B. Sheinin, Ph.D.
Philip D. Walson, M.D.

Drug Information Division Advisory Panels

Members who serve as Chairs are listed first.

The information presented in this text represents an ongoing review of the drugs contained herein and represents a consensus of various viewpoints expressed. The individuals listed below have

served on the USP Advisory Panels for the
1993–1994 revision period and have contributed to
the development of the 1995 USP DI database.
Such listing does not imply that these individuals
have reviewed all of the material in this text or
that they individually agree with all statements
contained herein.

Anesthesiology

Paul F. White, Ph.D., M.D., *Chair*, Dallas, TX; Eu-
gene Y. Cheng, M.D., Milwaukee, WI; Charles
J. Coté, M.D., Chicago, IL; Robert Feinstein,
M.D., St. Louis, MO; Peter S.A. Glass, M.D.,
Durham, NC; Michael B. Howie, M.D., Colum-
bus, OH; Beverly A. Krause, C.R.N.A., M.S., St.
Louis, MO; Carl Lynch, III, M.D., Ph.D., Char-
lottesville, VA; Carl Rosow, M.D., Ph.D., Bos-
ton, MA; Peter S. Sebel, M.B., Ph.D., Atlanta,
GA; Walter L. Way, M.D., Greenbrae, CA; Mat-
thew B. Weinger, M.D., San Diego, CA; Richard
Weiskopf, M.D., San Francisco, CA; David H.
Wong, Pharm.D., M.D., Long Beach, CA

Cardiovascular and Renal Drugs

Burton E. Sobel, M.D., *Chair*, St. Louis, MO; Wil-
liam P. Baker, M.D., Ph.D., Bethesda, MD; Nils
U. Bang, M.D., Indianapolis, IN; Emmanuel L.
Bravo, M.D., Cleveland, OH; Mary Jo Burgess,
M.D., Salt Lake City, UT; James H. Chesebro,
M.D., Boston, MA; Peter Corr, Ph.D., St. Louis,
MO; Dwain L. Eckberg, M.D., Richmond, VA;
Ruth Eshleman, Ph.D., W. Kingston, RI; William
H. Frishman, M.D., Bronx, NY; Edward D.
Frohlich, M.D., New Orleans, LA; Martha Hill,
Ph.D., R.N., Baltimore, MD; Norman M. Kaplan,
M.D., Dallas, TX; Michael Lesch, M.D., Detroit,
MI; Manuel Martinez-Maldonado, M.D., Deca-
tur, GA; Patrick A. McKee, M.D., Oklahoma

City, OK; Dan M. Roden, M.D., Nashville, TN; Michael R. Rosen, M.D., New York, NY; Jane Schultz, R.N., B.S.N., Rochester, MN; Robert L. Talbert, Pharm.D., San Antonio, TX; Raymond L. Woosley, M.D., Ph.D., Washington, DC

Clinical Immunology/Allergy/Rheumatology

Albert L. Sheffer, M.D., *Chair*, Boston, MA; John A. Anderson, M.D., Detroit, MI; Emil Bardana, Jr., M.D., Portland, OR; John Baum, M.D., Rochester, NY; Debra Danoff, M.D., Montreal, Quebec; Daniel G. de Jesus, M.D., Ph.D., Vanier, Ontario; Elliott F. Ellis, M.D., Jacksonville, FL; Patricia A. Fraser, M.D., Boston, MA; Frederick E. Hargreave, M.D., Hamilton, Ontario; Evelyn V. Hess, M.D., Cincinnati, OH; Jean M. Jackson, M.D., Boston, MA; Stephen R. Kaplan, M.D., Buffalo, NY; Sandra M. Koehler, Milwaukee, WI; Richard A. Moscicki, M.D., Newton, MA; Shirley Murphy, M.D., Albuquerque, NM; Gary S. Rachelefsky, M.D., Los Angeles, CA; Robert E. Reisman, M.D., Buffalo, NY; Robert L. Rubin, Ph.D., La Jolla, CA; Daniel J. Stechschulte, M.D., Kansas City, KS; Virginia S. Taggert, Bethesda, MD; Joseph A. Tami, Pharm.D., San Antonio, TX; John H. Toogood, M.D., London, Ontario; Martin D. Valentine, M.D., Baltimore, MD; Michael Weinblatt, M.D., Boston, MA; Dennis Michael Williams, Pharm.D., Chapel Hill, NC; Stewart Wong, Ph.D., Annandale, VA

Clinical Toxicology/Substance Abuse

Theodore G. Tong, Pharm.D., *Chair*, Tucson, AZ; John Ambre, M.D., Ph.D., Chicago, IL; Usoa E. Busto, Pharm.D., Toronto, Ontario; Darryl Inaba, Pharm.D., San Francisco, CA; Edward P. Krenzelok, Pharm.D., Pittsburgh, PA; Michael Montagne, Ph.D., Boston, MA; Sven A. Normann, Pharm.D., Tampa, FL; Gary M. Oderda,

Pharm.D., Salt Lake City, UT; Paul Pentel, M.D., Minneapolis, MN; Rose Ann Soloway, R.N., Washington, DC; Daniel A. Spyker, M.D., Ph.D., Rockville, MD; Anthony R. Temple, M.D., Ft. Washington, PA; Anthony Tommasello, Pharm.D., Baltimore, MD; Joseph C. Veltri, Pharm.D., Salt Lake City, UT; William A. Watson, Pharm.D., Kansas City, MO

Consumer Interest/Health Education

Gordon D. Schiff, M.D., *Chair*, Chicago, IL; Michael J. Ackerman, Ph.D., Bethesda, MD; Barbara Aranda-Naranjo, R.N., San Antonio, TX; Frank J. Ascione, Pharm.D., Ph.D., Ann Arbor, MI; Judith I. Brown, Silver Spring, MD; Jose Camacho, Austin, TX; Margaret A. Charters, Ph.D., Syracuse, NY; Jennifer Cross, San Francisco, CA; William G. Harless, Ph.D., Bethesda, MD; Louis H. Kompare, Lake Buena Vista, FL; Margo Kroshus, R.N., B.S.N., Rochester, MN; Marilyn Lister, Wakefield, Quebec; Margaret Lueders, Seattle, WA; Frederick S. Mayer, R.Ph., M.P.H., Sausalito, CA; Nancy Milio, Ph.D., Chapel Hill, NC; Irving Rubin, Port Washington, NY; T. Donald Rucker, Ph.D., River Forest, IL; Stephen B. Soumerai, Sc.D., Boston, MA; Carol A. Vetter, Rockville, MD

Critical Care Medicine

Catherine M. MacLeod, M.D., *Chair*, Chicago, IL; William Banner, Jr., M.D., Salt Lake City, UT; Philip S. Barie, M.D., New York, NY; Thomas P. Bleck, M.D., Charlottesville, VA; Roger C. Bone, M.D., Toledo, OH; Susan S. Fish, Pharm.D., Boston, MA; Edgar R. Gonzalez, Pharm.D., Richmond, VA; Robert Gottesman, Rockville, MD; John W. Hoyt, M.D., Pittsburgh, PA; Sheldon A. Magder, M.D., Montreal, Quebec; Joseph E. Parrillo, M.D., Chicago, IL; Sharon Peters, M.D.,

St. John's, Newfoundland; Domenic A. Sica, M.D., Richmond, VA; Martin G. Tweeddale, M.B., Ph.D., Vancouver, British Columbia

Dentistry

Sebastian G. Ciancio, D.D.S., *Chair*, Buffalo, NY; Donald F. Adams, D.D.S., Portland, OR; Karen A. Baker, M.S. Pharm., Iowa City, IA; Stephen A. Cooper, D.M.D., Ph.D., Philadelphia, PA; Frederick A. Curro, D.M.D., Ph.D., Jersey City, NJ; Paul J. Desjardins, D.M.D., Ph.D., Newark, NJ; Tommy W. Gage, D.D.S., Ph.D., Dallas, TX; Stephen F. Goodman, D.D.S., New York, NY; Daniel A. Haas, D.D.S., Ph.D., Toronto, Ontario; Richard E. Hall, D.D.S., Ph.D., Buffalo, NY; Lireka P. Joseph, Dr.P.H., Rockville, MD; Janice Lieberman, Fort Lee, NJ; Laurie Lisowski, Lewiston, NY; Clarence L. Trummel, D.D.S., Ph.D., Farmington, CT; Joel M. Weaver, II, D.D.S., Ph.D., Columbus, OH; Clifford W. Whall, Jr., Ph.D., Chicago, IL; Raymond P. White, Jr., D.D.S., Ph.D., Chapel Hill, NC; Ray C. Williams, D.M.D., Boston, MA

Dermatology

Robert S. Stern, M.D., *Chair*, Boston, MA; Beatrice B. Abrams, Ph.D., Somerville, NJ; Richard D. Baughman, M.D., Hanover, NH; Michael Bigby, M.D., Boston, MA; Janice T. Chussil, R.N., M.S.N., Portland, OR; Stuart Maddin, M.D., Vancouver, British Columbia; Milton Orkin, M.D., Robbinsdale, MN; Neil H. Shear, M.D., Toronto, Ontario; Edgar Benton Smith, M.D., Galveston, TX; Dennis P. West, M.S. Pharm., Lincolnshire, IL; Gail M. Zimmerman, Portland, OR

Diagnostic Agents—Nonradioactive

Robert L. Siegle, M.D., *Chair*, San Antonio, TX; Kaizer Aziz, Ph.D., Rockville, MD; Robert C.

Brasch, M.D., San Francisco, CA; Nicholas Harry Malakis, M.D., Bethesda, MD; Robert F. Mattrey, M.D., San Diego, CA; James A. Nelson, M.D., Seattle, WA; Jovitas Skucas, M.D., Rochester, NY; Gerald L. Wolf, Ph.D., M.D., Charlestown, MA

Drug Information Science

James A. Visconti, Ph.D., *Chair*, Columbus, OH; Marie A. Abate, Pharm.D., Morgantown, WV; Ann B. Amerson, Pharm.D., Lexington, KY; Philip O. Anderson, Pharm.D., San Diego, CA; Danial E. Baker, Pharm.D., Spokane, WA; C. David Butler, Pharm.D., M.B.A., Naperville, IL; Linda L. Hart, Pharm.D., Saddle River, NJ; Edward J. Huth, M.D., Philadelphia, PA; John M. Kessler, Pharm.D., Chapel Hill, NC; R. David Lauper, Pharm.D., Emeryville, CA; Domingo R. Martinez, Pharm.D., Birmingham, AL; William F. McGhan, Pharm.D., Ph.D., Philadelphia, PA; John K. Murdoch, B.Sc.Phm., Toronto, Ontario; Kurt A. Proctor, Ph.D., Alexandria, VA; Arnauld F. Scafidi, M.D., M.P.H., Rockville, MD; John A. Scarlett, M.D., Austin, TX; Gary H. Smith, Pharm.D., Tucson, AZ; Dennis F. Thompson, Pharm.D., Oklahoma City, OK; William G. Troutman, Pharm.D., Albuquerque, NM; Lee A. Wanke, M.S., Houston, TX

Drug Utilization Review

Judith K. Jones, M.D., Ph.D., *Chair*, Arlington, VA; John F. Beary, III, M.D., Washington, DC; James L. Blackburn, Pharm.D., Saskatoon, Saskatchewan; Richard S. Blum, M.D., East Hills, NY; Amy Cooper-Outlaw, Pharm.D., Stone Mountain, GA; Joseph W. Cranston, Jr., Ph.D., Chicago, IL; W. Gary Erwin, Pharm.D., Philadelphia, PA; Jere E. Goyan, Ph.D., Saddle River, NJ; Duane M. Kirking, Ph.D., Ann Arbor, MI;

Karen E. Koch, Pharm.D., Tupelo, MS; Aida A. LeRoy, Pharm.D., Arlington, VA; Jerome Levine, M.D., Baltimore, MD; Richard W. Lindsay, M.D., Charlottesville, VA; M. Laurie Mashford, M.D., Melbourne, Victoria, Australia; Deborah M. Nadzam, R.N., Ph.D., Oakbrook Terrace, IL; William Z. Potter, M.D., Ph.D., Bethesda, MD; Louise R. Rodriquez, M.S., Washington, DC; Stephen P. Spielberg, M.D., Ph.D., West Point, PA; Suzan M. Streichenwein, M.D., Houston, TX; Brian L. Strom, M.D., Philadelphia, PA; Michael Weintraub, M.D., Rockville, MD; Antonio Carlos Zanini, M.D., Ph.D., São Paulo, Brazil

Endocrinology

Maria I. New, M.D., *Chair*, New York, NY; Ronald D. Brown, M.D., Oklahoma City, OK; R. Keith Campbell, Pharm.D., Pullman, WA; David S. Cooper, M.D., Baltimore, MD; Betty J. Dong, Pharm.D., San Francisco, CA; Andrea Dunaif, M.D., New York, NY; Anke A. Ehrhardt, Ph.D., New York, NY; Nadir R. Farid, M.D., Durham, N.C.; John G. Haddad, Jr., M.D., Philadelphia, PA; Michael M. Kaplan, M.D., Southfield, MI; Harold E. Lebovitz, M.D., Brooklyn, NY; Marvin E. Levin, M.D., Chesterfield, MO; Marvin M. Lipman, M.D., Scarsdale, NY; Barbara J. Maschak-Carey, R.N., M.S.N., Philadelphia, PA; James C. Melby, M.D., Boston, MA; Walter J. Meyer, III, M.D., Galveston, TX; Rita Nemchik, R.N., M.S., C.D.E., Florence, NJ; Daniel A. Notterman, M.D., New York, NY; Ron Gershon Rosenfeld, M.D., Stanford, CA; Paul Saenger, M.D., Bronx, NY; Leonard Wartofsky, M.D., Washington, DC

Family Practice

Robert M. Guthrie, M.D., *Chair*, Columbus, OH; Jack A. Brose, D.O., Athens, OH; Jannet M. Car-

michael, Pharm.D., Reno, NV; Jacqueline A.
Chadwick, M.D., Scottsdale, AZ; Mark E. Cla-
sen, M.D., Ph.D., Dayton, OH; Lloyd P. Haskell,
M.D., West Borough, MA; Luis A. Izquierdo-
Mora, M.D., Rio Piedras, PR; Edward L. Langs-
ton, M.D., Houston, TX; Stephen T. O'Brien,
M.D., Enfield, CT; Charles D. Ponte, Pharm.D.,
Morgantown, WV; Jack M. Rosenberg,
Pharm.D., Ph.D., Brooklyn, NY; John F. Sang-
ster, M.D., London, Ontario; Theodore L. Yar-
boro, Sr., M.D., M.P.H., Sharon, PA

Gastroenterology
Gordon L. Klein, M.D., *Chair*, Galveston, TX; Karl
E. Anderson, M.D., Galveston, TX; William Bal-
istreri, M.D., Cincinnati, OH; Paul Bass, Ph.D.,
Madison, WI; Rosemary R. Berardi, Pharm.D.,
Ann Arbor, MI; Raymond F. Burk, M.D., Nash-
ville, TN; Thomas Q. Garvey, III, M.D., Poto-
mac, MD; Donald J. Glotzer, M.D., Boston, MA;
Flavio Habal, M.D., Toronto, Ontario; Paul E.
Hyman, M.D., Torrance, CA; Bernard Mehl,
D.P.S., New York, NY; William J. Snape, Jr.,
M.D., Torrance, CA; Ronald D. Soltis, M.D.,
Minneapolis, MN; C. Noel Williams, M.D., Hali-
fax, Nova Scotia; Hyman J. Zimmerman, M.D.,
Bethesda, MD

Geriatrics
Robert E. Vestal, M.D., *Chair*, Boise, ID; Darrell R.
Abernethy, M.D., Washington, DC; William B.
Abrams, M.D., West Point, PA; Jerry Avorn,
M.D., Boston, MA; Robert A. Blouin, Pharm.D.,
Lexington, KY; S. George Carruthers, M.D., Hal-
ifax, Nova Scotia; Lynn E. Chaitovitz, Rockville,
MD; Terry Fulmer, R.N., Ph.D., New York, NY;
Philip P. Gerbino, Pharm.D., Philadelphia, PA;
Pearl S. German, Sc.D., Baltimore, MD; David J.
Greenblatt, M.D., Boston, MA; Martin D.

Higbee, Pharm.D., Tucson, AZ; Brian B. Hoffman, M.D., Palo Alto, CA; J. Edward Jackson, M.D., San Diego, CA; Joseph V. Levy, Ph.D., San Francisco, CA; Paul A. Mitenko, M.D., FRCPC, Nanaimo, British Columbia; John E. Morley, M.B., B.Ch., St. Louis, MO; Jay Roberts, Ph.D., Philadelphia, PA; Louis J. Rubenstein, R.Ph., Alexandria, VA; Janice B. Schwartz, M.D., San Francisco, CA; Alexander M.M. Shepherd, M.D., San Antonio, TX; William Simonson, Pharm.D., Portland, OR; Daniel S. Sitar, Ph.D., Winnipeg, Manitoba; Mary K. Walker, R.N., Ph.D., Lexington, KY; Alastair J. J. Wood, M.D., Nashville, TN

Hematologic and Neoplastic Disease

John W. Yarbro, M.D., Ph.D., *Chair*, Springfield, IL; Joseph S. Bailes, M.D., McAllen, TX; Laurence H. Baker, D.O., Ann Arbor, MI; Barbara D. Blumberg-Carnes, Albuquerque, NM; Helene G. Brown, B.S., Los Angeles, CA; Nora L. Burnham, Pharm.D., Princeton, NJ; William J. Dana, Pharm.D., Houston, TX; Connie Henke-Yarbro, R.N., B.S.N., Springfield, IL; William H. Hryniuk, M.D., San Diego, CA; B. J. Kennedy, M.D., Minneapolis, MN; Barnett Kramer, M.D., Rockville, MD; Michael J. Mastrangelo, M.D., Philadelphia, PA; David S. Rosenthal, M.D., Cambridge, MA; Richard L. Schilsky, M.D., Chicago, IL; Rowena N. Schwartz, Pharm.D., Pittsburgh, PA; Roy L. Silverstein, M.D., New York, NY; Samuel G. Taylor, IV, M.D., Chicago, IL; Raymond B. Weiss, M.D., Washington, DC

Infectious Disease Therapy

Donald Kaye, M.D., *Chair*, Philadelphia, PA; Robert Austrian, M.D., Philadelphia, PA; C. Glenn Cobbs, M.D., Birmingham, AL; Joseph W. Cranston, Jr., Ph.D., Chicago, IL; John J. Dennehy,

M.D., Danville, PA; Courtney V. Fletcher,
Pharm. D., Minneapolis, MN; Earl H. Freimer,
M.D., Toledo, OH; Marc LeBel, Pharm.D., Que-
bec, Quebec; John D. Nelson, M.D., Dallas, TX;
Lindsay E. Nicolle, M.D., Winnipeg, Manitoba;
Alvin Novick, M.D., New Haven, CT; Charles
G. Prober, M.D., Stanford, CA; Douglas D. Rich-
man, M.D., San Diego, CA; Spotswood L.
Spruance, M.D., Salt Lake City, UT; Roy T.
Steigbigel, M.D., Stony Brook, NY; Paul F.
Wehrle, M.D., San Clemente, CA

International Health
Rosalyn C. King, Pharm.D., M.P.H., *Chair*, Silver
Spring, MD; Walter M. Batts, Rockville, MD;
Eugenie Brown, Pharm.D., Kingston, Jamaica;
Alan Cheung, Pharm.D., M.P.H., Washington,
DC; Mary Couper, M.D., Geneva, Switzerland;
Gabriel Daniel, Washington, DC; S. Albert Ed-
wards, Pharm.D., Lincolnshire, IL; Enrique
Fefer, Ph.D., Washington, DC; Peter H. M. Fon-
tilus, Curaçao, Netherlands Antilles; Gan Ee
Kiang, Penang, Malaysia; Marcellus Grace,
Ph.D., New Orleans, LA; George B. Griffenha-
gen, Washington, DC; Margareta Helling-Borda,
Geneva, Switzerland; Thomas Langston, Silver
Spring, MD; Thomas Lapnet-Moustapha,
Yaounde, Cameroon; David Lee, B.A., M.D., Ar-
lington, VA; Aissatov Lo, Ka-Olack, Senegal;
Stuart M. MacLeod, M.D., Hamilton, Ontario;
Russell E. Morgan, Jr., Dr.P.H., Chevy Chase,
MD; David Ofori-Adjei, M.D., Accra, Ghana; S.
Ofosu-Amaah, M.D., New York, NY; James
Rankin, Arlington, VA; Olikoye Ransome-Kuti,
M.D., Lagos, Nigeria; Budiono Santoso, M.D.,
Ph.D., Yogyakarta, Indonesia; Carmen Selva,
Ph.D., Madrid, Spain; Valentin Vinogradov,
Moscow, Russia; Fela Viso-Gurovich, Mexico

City, Mexico; William B. Walsh, M.D., Chevy
Chase, MD; Lawrence C. Weaver, Ph.D., Minne-
apolis, MN; Albert I. Wertheimer, Ph.D., Glen
Allen, VA

Neurology

Stanley van den Noort, M.D., *Chair*, Irvine, CA;
William T. Beaver, M.D., Washington, DC; Eliz-
abeth U. Blalock, M.D., Anaheim, CA; James C.
Cloyd, Pharm.D., Minneapolis, MN; David M.
Dawson, M.D., West Roxbury, MA; Kevin Far-
rell, M.D., Vancouver, British Columbia; Kath-
leen M. Foley, M.D., New York, NY; Anthony E.
Lang, M.D., Toronto, Ontario; Ira T. Lott, M.D.,
Orange, CA; James R. Nelson, M.D., La Jolla,
CA; J. Kiffin Penry, M.D., Winston-Salem, NC;
Neil H. Raskin, M.D., San Francisco, CA; Alfred
J. Spiro, M.D., Bronx, NY; M. DiAnn Turek,
R.N., Holt, MI

Nursing Practice

Rosemary C. Polomano, R.N., M.S.N., *Chair*, Philadelphia, PA; Mecca S. Cranley, R.N., Ph.D., Buffalo, NY; Jan M. Ellerhorst-Ryan, R.N., M.S.N.,
Cincinnati, OH; Linda Felver, Ph.D., R.N., Port-
land, OR; Hector Hugo Gonzalez, R.N., Ph.D.,
San Antonio, TX; Mary Harper, R.N., Ph.D.,
Rockville, MD; Ada K. Jacox, R.N., Ph.D., Balti-
more, MD; Patricia Kummeth, R.N., M.S., Roch-
ester, MN; Ida M. Martinson, R.N., Ph.D., San
Francisco, CA; Carol P. Patton, R.N., Ph.D., J.D.,
Detroit, MI; Ginette A. Pepper, R.N., Ph.D., En-
glewood, CO; Geraldine A. Peterson, R.N.,
M.A., Potomac, MD; Linda C. Pugh, R.N.,
Ph.D., York, PA; Sharon S. Rising, R.N., C.N.M.,
Cheshire, CT; Marjorie Ann Spiro, R.N., B.S.,
C.S.N., Scarsdale, NY

Nutrition and Electrolytes

Robert D. Lindeman, M.D., *Chair*, Albuquerque,

NM; Hans Fisher, Ph.D., New Brunswick, NJ; Walter H. Glinsmann, M.D., Washington, DC; Helen Andrews Guthrie, M.S., Ph.D., State College, PA; Steven B. Heymsfield, M.D., New York, NY; K. N. Jeejeebhoy, M.D., Toronto, Ontario; Leslie M. Klevay, M.D., Grand Forks, ND; Linda S. Knox, M.S.N., Philadelphia, PA; Bonnie Liebman, M.S., Washington, DC; Sudesh K. Mahajan, M.D., Grosse Point Woods, MI; Craig J. McClain, M.D., Lexington, KY; Jay M. Mirtallo, M.S., Columbus, OH; Sohrab Mobarhan, M.D., Maywood, IL; Robert M. Russell, M.D., Boston, MA; Harold H. Sandstead, M.D., Galveston, TX; William J. Stone, M.D., Nashville, TN; Carlos A. Vaamonde, M.D., Miami, FL; Stanley Wallach, M.D., New York, NY

Obstetrics and Gynecology

Douglas D. Glover, M.D., *Chair*, Morgantown, WV; Rudi Ansbacher, M.D., Ann Arbor, MI; Florence Comite, M.D., New Haven, CT; James W. Daly, M.D., Columbia, MO; Marilynn C. Frederiksen, M.D., Chicago, IL; Charles B. Hammond, M.D., Durham, NC; Barbara A. Hayes, M.A., New Rochelle, NY; Art Jacknowitz, Pharm.D., Morgantown, WV; William J. Ledger, M.D., New York, NY; Andre-Marie Leroux, M.D., Ottawa, Ontario; William A. Nahhas, M.D., Dayton, OH; Warren N. Otterson, M.D., Shreveport, LA; Samuel A. Pasquale, M.D., New Brunswick, NJ; Johanna Perlmutter, M.D., Boston, MA; Robert W. Rebar, M.D., Cincinnati, OH; Richard H. Reindollar, M.D., Boston, MA; G. Millard Simmons, M.D., Morgantown, WV; J. Benjamin Younger, M.D., Birmingham, AL

Ophthalmology

Herbert E. Kaufman, M.D., *Chair*, New Orleans, LA; Steven R. Abel, Pharm.D., Indianapolis, IN;

Jules Baum, M.D., Boston, MA; Lee R. Duffner, M.D., Miami, FL; David L. Epstein, M.D., Durham, NC; Allan J. Flach, Pharm.D., M.D., Corte Madera, CA; Vincent H. L. Lee, Ph.D., Los Angeles, CA; Steven M. Podos, M.D., New York, NY; Kirk R. Wilhelmus, M.D., Houston, TX; Thom J. Zimmerman, M.D., Ph.D., Louisville, KY

Otorhinolaryngology

Leonard P. Rybak, M.D., Ph.D., *Chair*, Springfield, IL; Robert E. Brummett, Ph.D., Portland, OR; Robert A. Dobie, M.D., San Antonio, TX; Linda J. Gardiner, M.D., Fort Myers, FL; David Hilding, M.D., Price, UT; David B. Hom, M.D., Minneapolis, MN; Helen F. Krause, M.D., Pittsburgh, PA; Richard L. Mabry, M.D., Dallas, TX; Lawrence J. Marentette, M.D., Ann Arbor, MI; Robert A. Mickel, M.D., Ph.D., San Francisco, CA; Randal A. Otto, M.D., San Antonio, TX; Richard W. Waguespack, M.D., Birmingham, AL; William R. Wilson, M.D., Washington, DC

Parasitic Disease

Jay S. Keystone, M.D., *Chair*, Toronto, Ontario; Michele Barry, M.D., New Haven, CT; Frank J. Bia, M.D., M.P.H., Guilford, CT; David Botero, M.D., Medellín, Colombia; David O. Freedman, M.D., Birmingham, AL; Elaine C. Jong, M.D., Seattle, WA; Dennis D. Juranek, M.D., Atlanta, GA; Donald J. Krogstad, M.D., New Orleans, LA; Douglas W. MacPherson, M.D., Hamilton, Ontario; Edward K. Markell, M.D., Berkeley, CA; Theodore Nash, M.D., Bethesda, MD; Murray Wittner, M.D., Bronx, NY

Patient Counseling (Ad Hoc)

Frank J. Ascione, Pharm.D., Ph.D., *Chair*, Ann Arbor, MI; John E. Arradondo, M.D., Houston, TX; Candace Barnett, Atlanta, GA; Karin Bolte,

Washington, DC; Allan H. Bruckheim, M.D.,
Harrison, NY; Mark Clasen, M.D., Ph.D., Day-
ton, OH; Amy Cooper-Outlaw, Pharm.D., Stone
Mountain, GA; Frederick A. Curro, D.M.D.,
Ph.D., Jersey City, NJ; Robin DiMatteo, Ph.D.,
Riverside, CA; Diane B. Ginsburg, Austin, TX;
Denise Grimes, R.N., Jackson, MI; Richard Her-
rier, Tucson, AZ; Barry Kass, R.Ph., Boston, MA;
Thomas Kellenberger, Pharm.D., Montvale, NJ;
Alice Kimball, Darnestown, MD; Pat Kramer,
Bismarck, ND; Patti Kummeth, R.N., Rochester,
MN; Ken Leibowitz, Philadelphia, PA; Colleen
Lum Lung, R.N., Denver, CO; Louise Matte,
Quebec, Canada; Scotti Milley, Richmond, VA;
Constance Pavlides, R.N., D.N.Sc., Rockville,
MD; Lisa Tedesco, Ph.D., Ann Arbor, MI

Pediatric Anesthesiology (Ad Hoc)
Charles J. Coté, M.D., *Chair*, Chicago, IL; J. Michael
Badgwell, M.D., Lubbock, TX; Barbara Bran-
dom, M.D., Pittsburgh, PA; Ryan Cook, M.D.,
Pittsburgh, PA; John J. Downes, M.D., Philadel-
phia, PA; Dennis Fisher, M.D., San Francisco,
CA; John E. Forestner, M.D., Fort Worth, TX;
Helen W. Karl, M.D., Seattle, WA; Harry G. G.
Kingston, M.B., Portland, OR; Anne Marie
Lynn, M.D., Seattle, WA; Mark Shriner, M.D.,
Philadelphia, PA; Victoria Simpson, M.D.,
Ph.D., Denver, CO; Meb Watcha, M.D., St.
Louis, MO

Pediatrics
Philip D. Walson, M.D., *Chair*, Columbus, OH;
Susan Alpert, Ph.D., M.D., Rockville, MD; Jacob
V. Aranda, M.D., Ph.D., Montreal, Quebec;
Cheston M. Berlin, Jr., M.D., Hershey, PA;
Nancy Jo Braden, M.D., Phoenix, AZ; Patricia J.
Bush, Ph.D., Washington, DC; Marion J. Finkel,
M.D., Morris Township, NJ; George S.

Goldstein, M.D., Briarcliff Manor, NY; Ralph E. Kauffman, M.D., Detroit, MI; Gideon Koren, M.D., Toronto, Ontario; Joan M. Korth-Bradley, Pharm.D., Ph.D., Philadelphia, PA; Richard Leff, Pharm.D., Kansas City, KS; Carolyn Lund, R.N., M.S., San Francisco, CA; Wayne Snodgrass, M.D., Galveston, TX; Celia A. Viets, M.D., Ottawa, Canada; John T. Wilson, M.D., Shreveport, LA; Sumner J. Yaffe, M.D., Bethesda, MD; Karin E. Zenk, Pharm.D., Irvine, CA

Pharmacy Practice

Thomas P. Reinders, Pharm.D., *Chair*, Richmond, VA; Olya Duzey, M.S., Big Rapids, MI; Yves Gariepy, B.Sc.Pharm., Quebec, Quebec; Ned Heltzer, M.S., New Castle, DE; Lester S. Hosto, B.S., Little Rock, AR; Martin J. Jinks, Pharm.D., Pullman, WA; Frederick Klein, B.S., Montvale, NJ; Calvin H. Knowlton, Ph.D., Lumberton, NJ; Patricia A. Kramer, B.S., Bismarck, ND; Dennis McCallum, Pharm.D., Minneapolis, MN; Shirley P. McKee, B.S., Houston, TX; William A. McLean, Pharm.D., Ottawa, Ontario; Gladys Montañez, B.S., Santurce, PR; Donald L. Moore, B.S., Kokomo, IN; John E. Ogden, M.S., Washington, DC; Henry A. Palmer, Ph.D., Storrs, CT; Lorie G. Rice, B.A., M.P.H., San Francisco, CA; Mike R. Sather, M.S., Albuquerque, NM; Albert Sebok, B.S., Hudson, OH; William E. Smith, Pharm.D., Ph.D., Boston, MA; Susan East Torrico, B.S., Orlando, FL; J. Richard Wuest, Pharm.D., Cincinnati, OH; Glenn Y. Yokoyama, Pharm.D., Pasadena, CA

Psychiatric Disease

Burton J. Goldstein, M.D., *Chair*, Williams Island, FL; Magda Campbell, M.D., New York, NY; Alex A. Cardoni, M.S. Pharm., Hartford, CT; James L. Claghorn, M.D., Houston, TX; N. Mi-

chael Davis, M.S., Miami, FL; Larry Ereshefsky,
Pharm.D., San Antonio, TX; W. Edwin Fann,
M.D., Houston, TX; Alan J. Gelenberg, M.D.,
Tucson, AZ; Tracy R. Gordy, M.D., Austin, TX;
Paul Grof, M.D., Ottawa, Ontario; Russell T.
Joffe, M.D., Toronto, Ontario; Nathan Rawls,
Pharm.D., Memphis, TN; Ruth Robinson, Saska-
toon, Saskatchewan; Matthew V. Rudorfer,
M.D., Rockville, MD; Karen A. Theesen,
Pharm.D., Omaha, NE

Pulmonary Disease
Harold S. Nelson, M.D., *Chair*, Denver, CO; Rich-
ard C. Ahrens, M.D., Iowa City, IA; Eugene R.
Bleecker, M.D., Baltimore, MD; William W.
Busse, M.D., Madison, WI; Christopher Fanta,
M.D., Boston, MA; Mary K. Garcia, R.N., Sug-
arland, TX; Nicholas Gross, M.D., Hines, IL;
Leslie Hendeles, Pharm.D., Gainesville, FL; El-
liot Israel, M.D., Boston, MA; Susan Janson-
Bjerklie, R.N., Ph.D., San Francisco, CA; John
W. Jenne, M.D., Hines, IL; H. William Kelly,
Pharm.D., Albuquerque, NM; James P. Kemp,
M.D., San Diego, CA; Henry Levison, M.D., To-
ronto, Ontario; Gail Shapiro, M.D., Seattle, WA;
Stanley J. Szefler, M.D., Denver, CO

Radiopharmaceuticals
Carol S. Marcus, Ph.D., M.D., *Chair*, Torrance, CA;
Capt. William H. Briner, B.S., Durham, NC;
Ronald J. Callahan, Ph.D., Boston, MA; Janet F.
Eary, M.D., Seattle, WA; Joanna S. Fowler,
Ph.D., Upton, NY; David L. Gilday, M.D., To-
ronto, Ontario; David A. Goodwin, M.D., Palo
Alto, CA; David L. Laven, N.Ph., C.R.Ph.,
FASCP, Bay Pines, FL; Andrea H. McGuire,
M.D., Des Moines, IA; Peter Paras, Ph.D., Rock-
ville, MD; Barry A. Siegel, M.D., St. Louis, MO;
Edward B. Silberstein, M.D., Cincinnati, OH;

Dennis P. Swanson, M.S., Pittsburgh, PA; Mathew L. Thakur, Ph.D., Philadelphia, PA; Henry N. Wellman, M.D., Indianapolis, IN

Surgical Drugs and Devices

Lary A. Robinson, M.D., *Chair*, Tampa, FL; Gregory Alexander, M.D., Rockville, MD; Norman D. Anderson, M.D., Baltimore, MD; Alan R. Dimick, M.D., Birmingham, AL; Jack Hirsh, M.D., Hamilton, Ontario; Manucher J. Javid, M.D., Madison, WI; Henry J. Mann, Pharm.D., Bloomington, MN; Kurt M. W. Niemann, M.D., Birmingham, AL; Robert P. Rapp, Pharm.D., Lexington, KY; Ronald Rubin, M.D., West Newton, MA

Urology

John A. Belis, M.D., *Chair*, Hershey, PA; Culley C. Carson, M.D., Chapel Hill, NC; Richard A. Cohen, M.D., Red Bank, NJ; B. J. Reid Czarapata, R.N., North Potomac, MD; Jean B. de Kernion, M.D., Los Angeles, CA; Warren Heston, Ph.D., New York, NY; Mark V. Jarowenko, M.D., Hershey, PA; Mary Lee, Pharm.D., Chicago, IL; Marguerite C. Lippert, M.D., Charlottesville, VA; Penelope A. Longhurst, Ph.D., Philadelphia, PA; Tom F. Lue, M.D., San Francisco, CA; Michael G. Mawhinney, Ph.D., Morgantown, WV; Martin G. McLoughlin, M.D., Vancouver, British Columbia; Randall G. Rowland, M.D., Ph.D., Indianapolis, IN; J. Patrick Spirnak, M.D., Cleveland, OH; William F. Tarry, M.D., Morgantown, WV; Keith N. Van Arsdalen, M.D., Philadelphia, PA

Veterinary Medicine

Lloyd E. Davis, D.V.M., Ph.D., *Chair*, Urbana, IL; Arthur L. Aronson, D.V.M., Ph.D., Raleigh, NC; Gordon W. Brumbaugh, D.V.M., Ph.D., College Station, TX; Peter Conlon, D.V.M., Ph.D.,

Guelph, Ontario; Gordon L. Coppoc, D.V.M., Ph.D., West Lafayette, IN; Sidney A. Ewing, D.V.M., Ph.D., Stillwater, OK; Stuart D. Forney, M.S., Fort Collins, CO; William G. Huber, D.V.M., Ph.D., Sun City West, AZ; Vernon Corey Langston, D.V.M., Ph.D., Mississippi State, MS; Mark G. Papich, D.V.M., Raleigh, NC; John W. Paul, D.V.M., Somerville, NJ; Thomas E. Powers, D.V.M., Ph.D., Columbus, OH; Charles R. Short, D.V.M., Ph.D., Baton Rouge, LA; Richard H. Teske, D.V.M., Ph.D., Rockville, MD; Jeffrey R. Wilcke, D.V.M., M.S., Blacksburg, VA

Drug Information Division Additional Contributors

The information presented in this text represents an ongoing review of the drugs contained herein and represents a consensus of various viewpoints expressed. In addition to the individuals listed below, many schools, associations, pharmaceutical companies, and governmental agencies have provided comment or otherwise contributed to the development of the 1995 USP DI database. Such listing does not imply that these individuals have reviewed all of the material in this text or that they individually agree with all statements contained herein.

Donald I. Abrams, M.D., San Francisco, CA
Jonathan Abrams, M.D., Albuquerque, NM
Bruce H. Ackerman, Pharm.D., Philadelphia, PA

N. Franklin Adkinson, M.D., Baltimore, MD
Allen C. Alfrey, M.D., Denver, CO
Joanne Allard, M.D., Toronto, Ontario, Canada
Carmen Allegra, M.D., Bethesda, MD
Mike Apley, D.V.M., Greeley, CO
Martin Bacon, M.D., Bethesda, MD
José M. Ballester, M.D., La Habana, Cuba
Rick Barbarash, Pharm.D., St. Louis, MO
Patsy Barnett, Pharm.D., Birmingham, AL
LuAnne Barron, Birmingham, AL
Robert W. Beightol, Pharm.D., Roanoke, VA
William Bell, M.D., Baltimore, MD
Gladys Bendahan Barchilón, Barcelona, Spain
Patricia Bennett, B.S.Pharm., Cincinnati, OH
David L. Benowitz, M.D., San Francisco, CA
Byron S. Berlin, M.D., Lansing, MI
Frederick A. Berry, M.D., Charlottesville, VA
Ernest Beutler, M.D., La Jolla, CA
Christine A. Bezouska, M.D., Morgantown, WV
S. Bruce Binder, M.D., Ph.D., Dayton, OH
Martin Black, M.D., Philadelphia, PA
Laura Boehnke, Pharm.D., Houston, TX
Halcy Bohen, Ph.D., Washington, DC
Wayne E. Bradley, Duluth, GA
Michael Brady, M.D., Columbus, OH
Edward L. Braud, M.D., Springfield, IL
Robert E. Braun, D.D.S., Buffalo, NY
Kenneth Bridges, M.D., Boston, MA
Paul J. Brown, M.D., Bedford, NH
Louis Buttino, Jr., M.D., Dayton, OH
Wesley G. Byerly, Pharm.D., Winston-Salem, NC
Karim A. Calis, Pharm.D., Bethesda, MD
Mary E. Carman, Ottawa, Ontario
Charles C.J. Carpenter, M.D., Providence, RI
Peggy Carver, M.D., Ann Arbor, MI
Marcel Casavant, M.D., Columbus, OH
Bruce A. Chabner, M.D., Bethesda, MD
Erin S. Champagne, D.V.M., Blacksburg, VA

Chih Wen Chang, Pharm.D., Maywood, IL
Te-Wen Chang, M.D., Boston, MA
Kenneth R. Chapman, M.D., Toronto, Ontario, Canada
Bruce D. Cheson, M.D., Bethesda, MD
Henry Chilton, Pharm.D., Winston-Salem, NC
Frank Chytil, Ph.D., Nashville, TN
Scott B. Citino, D.V.M., Yulee, FL
Cyril R. Clarke, Ph.D., Stillwater, OK
Jackson Como, M.D., Birmingham, AL
Betsy Jane Cooper, M.D., Washington, DC
James W. Cooper, Ph.D., Athens, GA
Deborah Cotton, M.D., Boston, MA
Fred F. Cowan, Ph.D., Portland, OR
Donald W. Cox, M.D., Morgantown, WV
Mark V. Crisman, D.V.M., Blacksburg, VA
Craig Darby, R.Ph., Twinsburg, OH
Michael Davidson, D.V.M., Raleigh, NC
Ann J. Davis, M.D., Boston, MA
Janet Davis, M.D., Miami, FL
Ken Davis, M.D., New York, NY
Thomas D. DeCillis, North Port, FL
Carel P. de Haseth, Ph.D., Netherland Antilles
Daniel Deykin, M.D., Boston, MA
Nick Diamant, M.D., Toronto, Ontario, Canada
Annette Dickinson, Ph.D., Washington, DC
Barry D. Dickinson, Ph.D., Chicago, IL
Christine Z. Dickinson, M.D., Royal Oak, MI
John B. DiMarco, M.D., Ph.D., Charlottesville, VA
James E. Doherty, M.D., Little Rock, AR
Donald C. Doll, M.D., Columbia, MO
Jerry Dolovich, M.D., Hamilton, Ontario, Canada
R. Gordon Douglas, M.D., Rahway, NJ
Ed Drea, Pharm.D., Phoenix, AZ
Bonnie Driggers, R.N., Portland, OR
Marion Dugdale, M.D., Memphis, TN
Carol Duncan, R.N., Portland, OR
Suzanne Eastman, M.S., R.Ph., Columbus, OH

John E. Edwards, Jr., M.D., Torrance, CA
Robert Edwards, Pharm.D., Columbus, OH
Lawrence H. Einhorn, M.D., Indianapolis, IN
Augustin Escalante, M.D., Downey, CA
Gary Euler, Dr.P.H., Atlanta, GA
William Fant, Pharm.D., Cincinnati, OH
Martin N. Farlow, M.D., Indianapolis, IN
R. Edward Faught, M.D., Birmingham, AL
David S. Fedson, M.D., Charlottesville, VA
John P. Feighner, La Mesa, CA
James M. Ferguson, M.D., Salt Lake City, UT
Paul Ferrell, M.D., Bethesda, MD
Anne Gilbert Feuer, R.Ph., Cincinnati, OH
Suzanne Fields, Pharm.D., San Antonio, TX
J.R. Fontilus, M.D., Netherland Antilles
Tammy Fox, R.Ph., Fairfield, OH
Charles W. Francis, M.D., Rochester, NY
Ruth Francis-Floyd, D.V.M., Gainesville, FL
Rudolph M. Franklin, M.D., New Orleans, LA
H. H. Frey, Berlin, Germany
Dorothy Friedberg, M.D., New York, NY
Alan Friedman, M.D., New York, NY
José P.B. Gallardo, R.Ph., Iowa City, IA
Gloria Garber, R.Ph., Cincinnati, OH
Arthur Garson, M.D., Durham, NC
S. Gauthier, M.D., Montreal, PQ, Canada
Edward Genton, M.D., New Orleans, LA
Anne A. Gershon, M.D., New York, NY
Larry N. Gever, Pharm.D., Cranbury, NJ
Michael J. Glade, Ph.D., Chicago, IL
Charles J. Glueck, M.D., Cincinnati, OH
Maryanne Godlewski-Vagnini, R.Ph.,
  Brooklyn, NY
Lewis Goldfrank, M.D., New York, NY
J. Max Goodson, D.D.S., Ph.D., Boston, MA
Fred Gordin, M.D., Washington, DC
John D. Grabenstein, M.S., Fort Sam Houston, TX
Roni Grad, M.D., Albuquerque, NM

Nina M. Graves, Pharm.D., Minneapolis, MN
Terri Graves Davidson, Pharm.D., Atlanta, GA
David Green, M.D., Chicago, IL
Harry Green, M.D., Evansville, IN
Martin D. Green, M.D., Rockville, MD
Philip C. Greig, M.D., Durham, NC
Vincent Habiyambere, M.D., Geneva, Switzerland
Angela M. Hadbavny, Pharm.D., Pittsburgh, PA
Benjamin F. Hammond, D.D.S., Ph.D., Philadelphia, PA
Kenneth R. Hande, M.D., Nashville, TN
Edward A. Hartshorn, Ph.D., League City, TX
Robert C. Hastings, M.D., Carville, LA
William E. Hathaway, Denver, CO
Frederick G. Hayden, M.D., Charlottesville, VA
Cleopatra L. Hazel, Pharm.D., Netherland Antilles
Murk-Hein Heinemann, M.D., New York, NY
Peter Hellyer, D.V.M., Raleigh, NC
Bryan N. Henderson, II, D.D.S., Dallas, TX
William Herbert, M.D., Durham, NC
Barbara Herwaldt, M.D., Atlanta, GA
Monto Ho, M.D., Pittsburgh, PA
Vincent C. Ho, M.D., British Columbia, Canada
M.E. Hoar, Springfield, MA
Robert Hodgeman, M.S., R.Ph., Cincinnati, OH
Gary N. Holland, M.D., Los Angeles, CA
Richard A. Holmes, M.D., Columbia, MO
William Hopkins, Pharm.D., Atlanta, GA
Richard B. Hornick, M.D., Orlando, FL
Raymond W. Houde, M.D., New York, NY
Colin W. Howden, M.D., Columbia, SC
Walter T. Hughes, M.D., Memphis, TN
B. Thomas Hutchinson, M.D., Boston, MA
John Iazzetta, Pharm.D., Toronto, Ontario, Canada
Rodney D. Ice, Ph.D., Atlanta, GA
Frederick Jacobsen, M.D., Washington, DC
Mark Jacobson, M.D., San Francisco, CA
Robert Jacobson, M.D., Carville, LA

Ann L. Janer, M.S., Auburn, AL
Janet P. Jaramilla, Pharm.D., Chicago, IL
James W. Jefferson, M.D., Madison, WI
Alan Jenkins, M.D., Charlottesville, VA
Leslye Johnson, Ph.D., Bethesda, MD
Joseph L. Jorizzo, M.D., Winston-Salem, NC
Gunnar Juliusson, M.D., Ph.D., Huddinge, Sweden
Hugh F. Kabat, Ph.D., Albuquerque, NM
James Kahn, M.D., San Francisco, CA
Alan Kanada, Pharm.D., Denver, CO
John J. Kavanagh, M.D., Houston, TX
Michael J. Keating, M.D., Houston, TX
Michael Kelley, M.D., Columbus, OH
David C. Kem, M.D., Oklahoma City, OK
N. David Kennedy, R.Ph., Washington, DC
Joseph M. Khoury, M.D., Bethesda, MD
Agnes V. Klein, M.D., Vanier, Ontario
Anne Klibanski, M.D., Boston, MA
Sandra Knowles, B.Pharm., Toronto, Ontario,
  Canada
John Koepke, Pharm.D., Columbus, OH
Joseph A. Kovacs, M.D., Bethesda, MD
Paul A. Krusinski, M.D., Burlington, VT
Paul B. Kuehn, Ph.D., Woodinville, WA
R.W. Kuncl, M.D., Baltimore, MD
Thomas L. Kurt, M.D., Dallas, TX
Lyle Laird, Pharm.D., San Antonio, TX
John S. Lambert, M.D., Rochester, NY
John R. LaMontagne, Bethesda, MD
Michael Lange, M.D., New York, NY
Victor J. Lanzotti, M.D., Springfield, IL
P. Reed Larsen, M.D., Boston, MA
Eugene Laska, M.D., Orangeburg, NY
Oscar L. Laskin, M.D., East Hanover, NJ
John Laszlo, M.D., Atlanta, GA
Belle Lee, Pharm.D., San Francisco, CA
Ilo E. Leppik, M.D., Minneapolis, MN
Raymond Levy, London, England

Richard A. Lewis, M.D., Houston, TX
William Lieber, M.D., Waterbury, CT
Charles Liebow, II, D.D.S., Ph.D., Buffalo, NY
Christopher D. Lind, M.D., Nashville, TN
Charles H. Livengood, III, M.D., Durham, NC
Don M. Long, M.D., Ph.D., Baltimore, MD
Julio R. Lopez, M.D., Martinez, CA
Colleen Lum Lung, R.N., Denver, CO
Howard I. Maibach, M.D., San Francisco, CA
Marilyn Manco-Johnson, Denver, CO
Victor J. Marder, M.D., Rochester, NY
Joseph E. Margarone, II, D.D.S., Buffalo, NY
Maurie Markman, M.D., Cleveland, OH
Jon Markovitz, M.D., Phoenix, AZ
William C. Matthews, M.D., San Diego, CA
Harry R. Maxon, III, M.D., Cincinnati, OH
Alice Lorraine McAfee, Pharm.D., San Pedro, CA
Lisa Y. McDonald, Pharm.D., Emeryville, CA
Norman L. McElroy, San Jose, CA
Charles McGrath, D.V.M., Blacksburg, VA
Ross E. McKinney, M.D., Durham, NC
Anne McNulty, M.D., Waterbury, CT
Wallace B. Mendelson, M.D., Cleveland, OH
Dean D. Metcalfe, M.D., Bethesda, MD
Donald Miller, Pharm.D., Fargo, ND
John Mills, M.D., Fairfield, Victoria, Australia
Joel S. Mindel, M.D., Ph.D., New York, NY
Bernard L. Mirkin, M.D., Chicago, IL
Janet L. Mitchell, M.D., New York, NY
John R. Modlin, M.D., Hanover, NH
C. Craig Moldenhauer, M.D., San Diego, CA
Garreth A. Moore, Blacksburg, VA
Mary E. Mortensen, M.D., Columbus, OH
Robyn Mueller, R.Ph., Cincinnati, OH
R.I. Ogilvie, M.D., Toronto, Ontario
Linda K. Ohri, Pharm.D., Omaha, NE
James M. Oleske, M.D., Newark, NJ
Robert O'Mara, M.D., Rochester, NY

Michael J. O'Neill, R.Ph., Twinsburg, OH
Walter A. Orenstein, M.D., Atlanta, GA
James R. Oster, M.D., Miami, FL
Judith M. Ozbun, R.Ph., M.S., Fargo, ND
David C. Pang, Ph.D., Chicago, IL
Michael F. Para, M.D., Columbus, OH
Satyapal R. Pareddy, B.Pharm., Brooklyn, NY
Robert C. Park, M.D., Washington, DC
William W. Parmly, M.D., San Francisco, CA
Albert Patterson, Hines, IL
James A. Pederson, M.D., Oklahoma City, OK
Ronald Peterson, M.D., Ph.D., Rochester, MN
Melenie Petropoulos, R.Ph., Twinsburg, OH
Lawrence D. Piro, M.D., La Jolla, CA
Philip A. Pizzo, M.D., Bethesda, MD
Christopher V. Plowe, M.D., Bethesda, MD
Therese Poirier, Pharm.D., Pittsburgh, PA
Michael A. Polis, M.D., Bethesda, MD
James A. Ponto, R.Ph., Iowa City, IA
Carol M. Proudfit, Ph.D., Chicago, IL
Nixa Ramos, Arecibo, Puerto Rico
Norbert P. Rapoza, Ph.D., Chicago, IL
Gary Raskob, M.Sc., Oklahoma City, OK
Terry D. Rees, D.D.S., Dallas, TX
Alfred J. Remillard, Pharm.D., Saskatoon, Saskatchewan, Canada
Robert Roberts, M.D., Houston, TX
David Robertson, M.D., Nashville, TN
Daniel C. Robinson, Pharm.D., Los Angeles, CA
John E. Roney, R.Ph., Cincinnati, OH
Jeff Rosner, R.Ph., Twinsburg, OH
Douglas S. Ross, M.D., Boston, MA
Phillip J. Rubin, M.D., Phoenix, AZ
Michael S. Saag, M.D., Birmingham, AL
Henry S. Sacks, Ph.D., M.D., New York, NY
Sharon Safrin, M.D., San Francisco, CA
Evelyn Salerno, Pharm.D., Hialeah, FL
Hugh A. Sampson, Jr., M.D., Baltimore, MD

Subbiah Sangiah, D.V.M., Ph.D., Stillwater, OK
Victor M. Santana, Memphis, TN
Belinda Sartor, M.D., Shreveport, LA
Donald C. Sawyer, East Lansing, MI
Elliot Schecter, M.D., Oklahoma City, OK
Udo P. Schmiedl, M.D., Ph.D., Seattle, WA
Gabriel Schmunis, M.D., Washington, DC
Steven M. Schnittman, M.D., Rockville, MD
George Schuster, M.D., Augusta, GA
Stephen Schuster, M.D., Philadelphia, PA
Dorothy Schwartz-Porsche, Berlin, Germany
Douglas A. Sears, Tenafly, NJ
Jerome Seidenfeld, Ph.D., Chicago, IL
Charles F. Seifert, Pharm.D., Oklahoma City, OK
Allen Shaughnessy, Pharm.D., Harrisburg, PA
Donald J. Sherrard, M.D., Seattle, WA
Yvonne M. Shevchuk, Pharm.D., Saskatoon, Saskatchewan, Canada
Harold M. Silverman, Pharm.D., Silver Spring, MD
Irv Siven, M.D., New York, NY
Barry H. Smith, M.D., Ph.D., New York, NY
Dance Smith, Pharm.D., Ft. Steilacoom, WA
Geralynn B. Smith, M.S., Detroit, MI
John R. Smith, M.S., Ph.D., Portland, OR
Steven J. Smith, Ph.D., Chicago, IL
Elliott M. Sogol, Ph.D., Research Triangle Park, NC
Nicholas Soter, M.D., New York, NY
William Speliacy, M.D., Tampa, FL
Joan Stachnik, Chicago, IL
William Steers, M.D., Charlottesville, VA
John J. Stern, M.D., Philadelphia, PA
Irwin Strathman, M.D., Lutz, FL
Kris Strohbehn, M.D., Boston, MA
David Stuhr, Denver, CO
Alan Sugar, M.D., Boston, MA
Linda Gore Sutherland, Pharm.D., Laramie, WY
Sandra Tailor, Pharm.D., Toronto, Ontario, Canada
David A. Taylor, M.D., Morgantown, WV

Mary E. Teresi, Iowa City, IA
Cheryl Nunn Thompson, Chicago, IL
John C. Thurman, D.V.M., Urbana, IL
Roger C. Toffle, M.D., Morgantown, WV
Douglas M. Tollefsen, M.D., St. Louis, MO
Eric J. Topol, M.D., Ann Arbor, MI
Jayme Trott, Pharm.D., San Antonio, TX
Donald G. Vidt, M.D., Cleveland, OH
Richard Vogel, D.D.S., Newark, NJ
Georgia Vogelsang, M.D., Baltimore, MD
Paul A. Volberding, M.D., San Francisco, CA
Andrea Wall, R.Ph., Cincinnati, OH
William Warner, Ph.D., New York, NY
Michael Weber, M.D., Irvine, CA
Krisantha Weerasuriya, M.D., Geneva, Switzerland
G. John Weir, M.D., Marshfield, WI
Timothy E. Welty, Pharm.D., Cincinnati, OH
Stanford Wessler, M.D., Rye, NY
Carolyn Westhoff, New York, NY
John White, Pharm.D., Spokane, WA
Richard J. Whitley, M.D., Birmingham, AL
Catherine Wilfert, M.D., Durham, NC
Robert G. Wolfangel, Ph.D., St. Louis, MO
M. Michael Wolfe, M.D., Boston, MA
William Wonderlin, Ph.D., Morgantown, WV
Richard J. Wood, M.D., Boston, MA
Curtis Wright, M.D., Rockville, MD
Catharine Wuest, R.Ph., Cincinnati, OH
Robert Yarchoan, M.D., Bethesda, MD
John M. Zajecka, M.D., Chicago, IL
Stephanie Zarus, Pharm.D., Philadelphia, PA
Frederic J. Zucchero, M.A., R.Ph., Chesterfield, MO
Jane R. Zucker, Atlanta, GA

Headquarters Staff

DRUG INFORMATION DIVISION
Director: Keith W. Johnson
Assistant Director: Georgie M. Cathey
Administrative Staff: Jaime A. Ramirez *(Administrative Assistant)*, Albert Crucillo, Mayra L. Rios
Senior Drug Information Specialists: Sandra Lee Boyer, Nancy Lee Dashiell, Debra A. Edwards, Esther H. Klein *(Supervisor)*, Angela Méndez Mayo *(Spanish Publications Coordinator)*
Drug Information Specialists: Katherine M. Bennett, Joyce Carpenter, Ann Corken, Jymeann King, Doris Lee *(Supervisor)*, Robin Schermerhorn, Denise Seldon, Daniel W. Seyoum
Veterinary Drug Information Specialist: Amy Neal
Coordinator, Patient Counseling and Education Programs: Stacy M. Hartranft
Computer Applications: Richard Allen *(Programmer)*, Bernard G. Silverstein *(Computer Applications Specialist)*
Publications Development Staff: Diana M. Blais *(Manager)*, Anne M. Lawrence *(Associate)*, Dorothy Raymond *(Assistant)*, Darcy Schwartz *(Assistant)*
Library Services: Florence A. Hogan *(Manager)*, Terri Rikhy *(Assistant)*, Madeleine Welsch
Research Associate, International Programs: David D. Housley
Research Assistant: Annamarie J. Sibik
Consultants: Janet Elgert, Lourdes de Gonzalez, David W. Hughes, S. Ramakrishnan Iyer, Wanda Janicki, Kate Phelan, Marcelo Vernengo

Scholar in Residence: Patricia J. Bush, Georgetown University

Student Interns/Externs: Robyn Dubinsky, University of Missouri at Kansas City; Rachel Ellis, Nottingham University, England; Kevin Garey, Dalhousie University, Nova Scotia; Bereket Melaku, Howard University; Kavita Nair, University of Toledo; Ken Rogers, University of Arizona; Yván Sánchez-Huamaní, National University of Trujillo, Peru

Visiting Scholars: Giulia Cingolani, Rome, Italy; Elena Oshkalova, Moscow, Russian Federation; Svetlana Udotova, Moscow, Russian Federation

---

USP ADMINISTRATIVE STAFF

Executive Director: Jerome A. Halperin
Associate Executive Director: Joseph G. Valentino
Assistant Executive Director for Professional and Public Affairs: Jacqueline L. Eng
Director, Finance: Abe Brauner
Director, Operations: J. Robert Strang
Director, Personnel: Arlene Bloom
Director, Fulfillment/Facilities: Drew J. Lutz
Legal: Kim Keller (Staff Attorney), John Lindow (Associate Legal Counsel for Business Affairs), Colleen Ottoson (Staff Attorney)

DRUG STANDARDS DIVISION

Director: Lee T. Grady

Assistant Directors: Charles H. Barnstein *(Revision)*, Barbara B. Hubert *(Scientific Administration)*, Robert H. King *(Technical Services)*

Senior Scientists: Roger Dabbah, V. Srinivasan, William W. Wright

Scientists: Frank P. Barletta, Vivian A. Gray, W. Larry Paul

Senior Scientific Associate: Todd L. Cecil

Technical Editors: Ann K. Ferguson, Melissa M. Smith

Supervisor of Administration: Anju K. Malhotra

Support Staff: Patricia Barnhill, Glenna Etherton, Theresa H. Lee, Cecilia Luna, Maureen Rawson, Ernestene Williams

Drug Research and Testing Laboratory: Richard F. Lindauer *(Director)*

Hazard Communications: Linda Shear

Consultants: J. Joseph Belson, Zorach R. Glaser, Martin Golden, Aubrey S. Outschoorn

---

MARKETING

Vice-President, Marketing and Sales: Mark Sohasky

Category Manager: Joan April *(Drug and Therapeutic Information)*

Assistant Category Manager: Pam Nelson *(Patient Education)*

Senior Account Manager: Susan Williams *(Electronic Products)*

Account Managers: Charlotte McKamy, Mary Dougherty *(Electronic Products)*

Marketing Associate: Matthew Valleskey

PUBLICATION SERVICES

Managing Editors: A. V. Precup *(USP DI)*, Sandra Boynton *(USP-NF)*

Editorial Associates: *USP DI*—Ellen R. Loeb *(Senior Editorial Associate)*, Carol M. Griffin, Carol N. Hankin, Marie Kotomori, Harriet S. Nathanson, Ellen D. Smith, Barbara A. Visco; *USP-NF*—Jesusa D. Cordova *(Senior Editorial Associate)*, Ellen Elovitz, John Pahle, Margaret Kay Walshaw

USAN Staff: Carolyn A. Fleeger *(Editor)*, Gerilynne Seigneur

Typesetting Systems Coordinator: Jean E. Dale

Typesetting Staff: Susan L. Entwistle *(Supervisor)*, Donna Alie, Deborah R. Connelly, Lauren Taylor Davis, Deborah James, M. T. Samahon, Micheline Tranquille

Graphics: Cristy Gonzalez, Todd Hodges, Tia C. Morfessis, Greg Varhola

Word Processing: Barbara A. Bowman *(Supervisor)*, Frances Rampp, Susan Schartman, Jane Shulman

Also Contributing: Barbara Arnold, Proofreading; Brian Dillon and Paul Widem of Editech Services, Inc., Proofreading; Terri A. DeIuliis, Graphics; Michelle Thomas, Clerical Assistance.

PRACTITIONER REPORTING PROGRAMS

Assistant Executive Director for Practitioner Reporting Programs: Diane D. Cousins

Staff: Robin A. Baldwin, Shawn C. Becker, Jean Canada, Alice C. Curtis, Ilze Mohseni, Joanne Pease, Susmita Samanta, Anne Paula Thompson, Mary Susan Zmuda

Members of the USPC
and the Institutions and
Organizations Represented
as of March 15, 1994

American Hospital Association: William R. Reid

American Medical Association: Joseph W. Cranston, Jr., Ph.D.

American Nurses Association: Linda Cronenwett, Ph.D., R.N., F.A.A.N.

American Pharmaceutical Association: Arthur H. Kibbe, Ph.D.

American Society for Clinical Pharmacology & Therapeutics: William J. Mroczek, M.D.

American Society of Consultant Pharmacists: Milton S. Moskowitz

American Society of Hospital Pharmacists: Charles E. Myers

American Society for Pharmacology and Experimental Therapeutics: Kenneth L. Dretchen

American Society for Quality Control: Anthony M. Carfagno

American Veterinary Medical Association: Lloyd Davis, D.V.M., Ph.D.

Animal Health Institute: Martin Terry, D.V.M., Ph.D.

Association of Food and Drug Officials: David R. Work, J.D.

Association of Official Analytical Chemists: Thomas Layloff, Jr.

Chemical Manufacturers Association: Andrew J. Schmitz, Jr. *(deceased)*

Cosmetic, Toiletry & Fragrance Association, Inc.: G.N. McEwen, Jr., Ph.D., J.D.

Council for Responsible Nutrition: Annette Dickinson, Ph.D.

Drug Information Association: Elizabeth B. D'Angelo, Ph.D.

Generic Pharmaceutical Industry Association: William F. Haddad

Health Industry Manufacturers Association: Dee Simons

National Association of Boards of Pharmacy: Carmen Catizone

National Association of Chain Drug Stores, Inc.: Saul Schneider

National Pharmaceutical Alliance: Christina F. Sizemore

National Wholesale Druggists' Association: Bruce R. Siecker, R.Ph., Ph.D.

Nonprescription Drug Manufacturers Association: R. William Soller, Ph.D.

Parenteral Drug Association, Inc.: Peter E. Manni, Ph.D.

Pharmaceutical Manufacturers Association: Maurice Q. Bectel

Other Organizations and Institutions

Alabama

Auburn University, School of Pharmacy: Kenneth N. Barker, Ph.D.

Samford University School of Pharmacy: H. Anthony McBride, Ph.D.

University of Alabama School of Medicine: Robert B. Diasio, M.D.

University of South Alabama, College of Medicine: Samuel J. Strada, Ph.D.

Medical Association of the State of Alabama: Paul A. Palmisano, M.D.

Alabama Pharmaceutical Association: Mitchel C. Rothholz

Alaska

Alaska Pharmaceutical Association: Jackie Warren, R.Ph.

Arizona

University of Arizona, College of Medicine: John D. Palmer, Ph.D., M.D.

University of Arizona, College of Pharmacy: Michael Mayersohn, Ph.D.

Arizona Pharmacy Association: Edward Armstrong

Arkansas

University of Arkansas for Medical Sciences, College of Pharmacy: Kenneth G. Nelson, Ph.D.

Arkansas Pharmacists Association: Norman Canterbury, P.D.

California

Loma Linda University Medical Center: Ralph Cutler, M.D.

Stanford University School of Medicine: Brian B. Hoffman, M.D.

University of California, Davis, School of Medicine: Larry Stark, Ph.D.

University of California, San Diego, School of Medicine: Harold J. Simon, M.D., Ph.D.

University of California, San Francisco, School of Medicine: Walter L. Way, M.D.

University of Southern California, School of Medicine: Wayne R. Bidlack, Ph.D.

University of California, San Francisco, School of Pharmacy: Richard H. Guy, Ph.D.

University of Southern California, School of Pharmacy: Robert T. Koda, Pharm.D., Ph.D.

University of the Pacific, School of Pharmacy: Alice Jean Matuszak, Ph.D.

California Pharmacists Association: Robert P. Marshall, Pharm.D.

Colorado

University of Colorado School of Pharmacy: Merrick Lee Shively, Ph.D.

Colorado Pharmacists Association: Thomas G. Arthur, R.Ph.

Connecticut

University of Connecticut, School of Medicine: Paul F. Davern

University of Connecticut, School of Pharmacy: Karl A. Nieforth, Ph.D.

Connecticut Pharmaceutical Association: Henry A. Palmer, Ph.D.

Delaware

Delaware Pharmaceutical Society: Charles J. O'Connor

Medical Society of Delaware: John M. Levinson, M.D.

District of Columbia

George Washington University: Janet Elgert-Madison, Pharm.D.

Georgetown University, School of Medicine: Arthur Raines, Ph.D.

Howard University, College of Medicine: Sonya K. Sobrian, Ph.D.

Howard University, College of Pharmacy & Pharmacal Sciences: Wendell T. Hill, Jr., Pharm.D.

Florida

Southeastern College of Pharmacy: William D. Hardigan, Ph.D.

University of Florida, College of Medicine: Thomas F. Muther, Ph.D.

University of Florida, College of Pharmacy: Michael A. Schwartz, Ph.D.

University of South Florida, College of Medicine: Joseph J. Krzanowski, Jr., Ph.D.

Florida Pharmacy Association: "Red" Camp

Georgia

Medical College of Georgia, School of Medicine: David W. Hawkins, Pharm.D.

Mercer University School of Medicine: W. Douglas Skelton, M.D.

Mercer University, Southern School of Pharmacy: Hewitt W. Matthews, Ph.D.

Morehouse School of Medicine: Ralph W. Trottier, Jr., Ph.D., J.D.

University of Georgia, College of Pharmacy: Stuart Feldman, Ph.D.

Medical Association of Georgia: E. D. Bransome, Jr., M.D.

Georgia Pharmaceutical Association, Inc.: Larry R. Braden

Idaho

Idaho State University, College of Pharmacy: Eugene I. Isaacson, Ph.D.

Idaho State Pharmaceutical Association: Doris Denney

Illinois

Chicago Medical School/University of Health Sciences: Velayudhan Nair, Ph.D., D.Sc.

Loyola University of Chicago, Stritch School of Medicine: Erwin Coyne, Ph.D.

Northwestern University Medical School: Marilynn C. Frederiksen, M.D.

Rush Medical College of Rush University: Paul G. Pierpaoli, M.S.

Southern Illinois University, School of Medicine: Leonard Rybak, M.D., Ph.D.

University of Chicago, Pritzker School of Medicine: Patrick T. Horn, M.D., Ph.D.

University of Illinois, College of Medicine: Marten M. Kernis, Ph.D.

University of Illinois, College of Pharmacy: Henri R. Manasse, Jr., Ph.D.

Chicago College of Pharmacy: David J. Slatkin, Ph.D.

Illinois Pharmacists Association: Ronald W. Gottrich

Illinois State Medical Society: Vincent A. Costanzo, Jr., M.D.

Indiana

Butler University, College of Pharmacy: Wagar H. Bhatti, Ph.D.

Purdue University, School of Pharmacy and Pharmacal Sciences: Garnet E. Peck, Ph.D.

Indiana State Medical Association: Edward Langston, R.Ph., M.D.

Iowa

Drake University, College of Pharmacy: Sidney L. Finn, Ph.D.

University of Iowa, College of Medicine: John E. Kasik, M.D., Ph.D.

University of Iowa, College of Pharmacy: Robert A. Wiley, Ph.D.

Iowa Pharmacists Association: Steve C. Firman, R.Ph.

Kansas

University of Kansas, School of Pharmacy: Prof. Christopher Riley

Kansas Pharmacists Association: Robert R. Williams

Kentucky

University of Kentucky, College of Medicine: John M. Carney, Ph.D.

University of Kentucky, College of Pharmacy: Patrick P. DeLuca, Ph.D.

University of Louisville, School of Medicine: Peter P. Rowell, Ph.D.

Kentucky Medical Association: Ellsworth C. Seeley, M.D.

Kentucky Pharmacists Association: Chester L. Parker, Pharm.D.

Louisiana

Louisiana State University School of Medicine in New Orleans: Paul L. Kirkendol, Ph.D.

Northeast Louisiana University, School of Pharmacy: William M. Bourn, Ph.D.

Tulane University, School of Medicine: Floyd R. Domer, Ph.D.

Xavier University of Louisiana: Barry A. Bleidt, Ph.D., R.Ph.

Louisiana State Medical Society: Henry W. Jolly, Jr., M.D.
Louisiana Pharmacists Association: Mona J. Davis

Maryland

Johns Hopkins University, School of Medicine: E. Robert Feroli, Jr., Pharm.D.
University of Maryland, School of Medicine: Edson X. Albuquerque, M.D., Ph.D.
Uniformed Services University of the Health Sciences, F. Edward Hebert School of Medicine: Louis R. Cantilena, Jr., M.D., Ph.D.
University of Maryland, Baltimore, School of Pharmacy: Larry L. Augsburger, Ph.D.
Medical and Chirurgical Faculty of the State of Maryland: Frederick Wilhelm, M.D.
Maryland Pharmacists Association: Nicholas C. Lykos, P.D.

Massachusetts

Boston University, School of Medicine: J. Worth Estes, M.D.
Harvard Medical School: Peter Goldman, M.D.
Massachusetts College of Pharmacy and Allied Health Sciences: David A. Williams, Ph.D.
Northeastern University, College of Pharmacy and Allied Health Professions: John L. Neumeyer, Ph.D.
Tufts University, School of Medicine: John Mazzullo, M.D.
University of Massachusetts Medical School: Brian Johnson, M.D.
Massachusetts Medical Society: Errol Green, M.D.

Michigan

Ferris State University, School of Pharmacy: Gerald W.A. Slywka, Ph.D.
Michigan State University, College of Human Medicine: John Penner, M.D.
University of Michigan, College of Pharmacy: Ara G. Paul, Ph.D.
University of Michigan Medical Center: Jeoffrey K. Stross, M.D.
Wayne State University, School of Medicine: Ralph E. Kauffman, M.D.
Wayne State University, College of Pharmacy and Allied Health Professions: Janardan B. Nagwekar, Ph.D.
Michigan Pharmacists Association: Patrick L. McKercher, Ph.D.

Minnesota

Mayo Medical School: James J. Lipsky, M.D.

University of Minnesota, College of Pharmacy: E. John Staba, Ph.D.

University of Minnesota Medical School, Minneapolis: Jack W. Miller, Ph.D.

Minnesota Medical Association: Harold Seim, M.D.

Minnesota Pharmacists Association: Arnold D. Delger

Mississippi

University of Mississippi, School of Medicine: James L. Achord, M.D.

University of Mississippi, School of Pharmacy: Robert W. Cleary, Ph.D.

Mississippi State Medical Association: Charles L. Mathews

Mississippi Pharmacists Association: Mike Kelly

Missouri

St. Louis College of Pharmacy: John W. Zuzack, Ph.D.

St. Louis University, School of Medicine: Alvin H. Gold, Ph.D.

University of Missouri, Columbia, School of Medicine: John W. Yarbro, M.D.

University of Missouri, Kansas City, School of Medicine: Paul Cuddy, Pharm.D.

University of Missouri, Kansas City, School of Pharmacy: Lester Chafetz, Ph.D.

Washington University, School of Medicine: H. Mitchell Perry, Jr., M.D.

Missouri Pharmaceutical Association: George L. Oestreich

Montana

The University of Montana, School of Pharmacy & Allied Health Sciences: David S. Forbes, Ph.D.

Nebraska

Creighton University, School of Medicine: Michael C. Makoid, Ph.D.

Creighton University School of Pharmacy and Allied Health Professions: Kenneth R. Keefner, Ph.D.

University of Nebraska, College of Medicine: Manuchair Ebadi, Ph.D.

University of Nebraska, College of Pharmacy: Clarence T. Ueda, Pharm.D., Ph.D.

Nebraska Pharmacists Association: Rex C. Higley, R.P.

Nevada
Nevada Pharmacists Association: Steven P. Bradford

New Hampshire
Dartmouth Medical School: James J. Kresel, Ph.D.
New Hampshire Pharmaceutical Association: William J. Lancaster, P.D.

New Jersey
University of Medicine and Dentistry of New Jersey, New Jersey Medical School: Sheldon B. Gertner, Ph.D.
Rutgers, The State University of New Jersey, College of Pharmacy: John L. Colaizzi, Ph.D.
Medical Society of New Jersey: Joseph N. Micale, M.D.
New Jersey Pharmaceutical Association: Stephen J. Csubak, Ph.D.

New Mexico
University of New Mexico, College of Pharmacy: William M. Hadley, Ph.D.
New Mexico Pharmaceutical Association: Hugh Kabat, Ph.D.

New York
Albert Einstein College of Medicine of Yeshiva University: Walter G. Levine, Ph.D.
City University of New York, Mt. Sinai School of Medicine: Joel S. Mindel, M.D., Ph.D.
Columbia University College of Physicians and Surgeons: Michael R. Rosen, M.D.
Cornell University Medical College: Lorraine J. Gudas, Ph.D.
Long Island University, Arnold and Marie Schwartz College of Pharmacy and Health Sciences: Jack M. Rosenberg, Ph.D.
New York Medical College: Mario A. Inchiosa, Jr., Ph.D.
New York University School of Medicine: Norman Altzuler, Ph.D.
State University of New York, Buffalo, School of Medicine: Robert J. McIsaac, Ph.D.
State University of New York, Buffalo, School of Pharmacy: Robert M. Cooper
State University of New York, Health Science Center, Syracuse: Oliver M. Brown, Ph.D.

St. John's University, College of Pharmacy and Allied Health Professions: Albert A. Belmonte, Ph.D.

Union University, Albany College of Pharmacy: David W. Newton, Ph.D.

University of Rochester, School of Medicine and Dentistry: Michael Weintraub, M.D., Ph.D.

Medical Society of the State of New York: Richard S. Blum, M.D.

Pharmaceutical Society of the State of New York: Bruce Moden

North Carolina

Bowman Gray School of Medicine, Wake Forest University: Jack W. Strandhoy, Ph.D.

Campbell University, School of Pharmacy: Antoine Al-Achi, Ph.D.

Duke University Medical Center: William J. Murray, M.D., Ph.D.

East Carolina University, School of Medicine: A-R.A. Abdel-Rahman, Ph.D.

University of North Carolina, Chapel Hill, School of Medicine: George Hatfield, Ph.D.

University of North Carolina, Chapel Hill, School of Pharmacy: Richard J. Kowalsky, Pharm.D.

North Carolina Pharmaceutical Association: George H. Co-colas, Ph.D.

North Carolina Medical Society: T. Reginald Harris, M.D.

North Dakota

University of North Dakota, School of Medicine: David W. Hein, Ph.D.

North Dakota State University, College of Pharmacy: William M. Henderson, Ph.D.

North Dakota Medical Association: Vernon E. Wagner

North Dakota Pharmaceutical Association: William H. Shelver, Ph.D.

Ohio

Case Western Reserve University, School of Medicine: Kenneth A. Scott, Ph.D.

Medical College of Ohio at Toledo: R. Douglas Wilkerson, Ph.D.

Northeastern Ohio University, College of Medicine: Ralph E. Berggren, M.D.

Ohio Northern University, College of Pharmacy: Joseph
   Theodore, Ph.D.
Ohio State University, College of Medicine: Robert
   Guthrie, M.D.
Ohio State University, College of Pharmacy: Michael C.
   Gerald, Ph.D.
University of Cincinnati, College of Medicine: Leonard T.
   Sigell, Ph.D.
University of Cincinnati, College of Pharmacy: Henry S.I.
   Tan, Ph.D.
University of Toledo, College of Pharmacy: Norman F. Bill-
   ups, Ph.D.
Wright State University, School of Medicine: John O. Lin-
   dower, M.D., Ph.D.
Ohio State Medical Association: Janet K. Bixel, M.D.
Ohio State Pharmaceutical Association: J. Richard Wuest,
   Pharm.D.

Oklahoma

University of Oklahoma College of Medicine: Ronald D.
   Brown, M.D.
*Southwestern Oklahoma State University, School of Phar-
   macy:* W. Steven Pray, Ph.D.
University of Oklahoma, College of Pharmacy: Loyd V.
   Allen, Jr., Ph.D.
Oklahoma State Medical Association: Clinton Nicholas
   Corder, M.D., Ph.D.
Oklahoma Pharmaceutical Association: Carl D. Lyons

Oregon

Oregon Health Sciences University, School of Medicine: Hall
   Downes, M.D., Ph.D.
Oregon State University, College of Pharmacy: Randall L.
   Vanderveen, Ph.D.

Pennsylvania

Duquesne University, School of Pharmacy: Lawrence H.
   Block, Ph.D.
Hahnemann University, School of Medicine: Vincent J.
   Zarro, M.D., Ph.D.
Medical College of Pennsylvania: Athole G. McNeil Ja-
   cobi, M.D.
Pennsylvania State University, College of Medicine: John D.
   Connor, Ph.D.

Philadelphia College of Pharmacy and Science: Alfonso R. Gennaro, Ph.D.

Temple University, School of Medicine: Ronald J. Tallarida, Ph.D.

Temple University, School of Pharmacy: Murray Tuckerman, Ph.D.

University of Pennsylvania, School of Medicine: Marilyn E. Hess, Ph.D.

University of Pittsburgh, School of Pharmacy: Terrence L. Schwinghammer, Pharm.D.

Pennsylvania Medical Society: Benjamin Calesnick, M.D.

Pennsylvania Pharmaceutical Association: Joseph A. Mosso, R.Ph.

Puerto Rico

Universidad Central del Caribe, School of Medicine: Jesús Santos-Martínez, Ph.D.

University of Puerto Rico, College of Pharmacy: Benjamin P. de Gracia, Ph.D.

University of Puerto Rico, School of Medicine: Walmor C. De Mello, M.D., Ph.D.

Rhode Island

Brown University Program in Medicine: Darrell R. Abernethy, M.D., Ph.D.

University of Rhode Island, College of Pharmacy: Thomas E. Needham, Ph.D.

South Carolina

Medical University of South Carolina, College of Medicine: Herman B. Daniell, Ph.D.

Medical University of South Carolina, College of Pharmacy: Paul J. Niebergall, Ph.D.

University of South Carolina, College of Pharmacy: Robert L. Beamer, Ph.D.

South Dakota

South Dakota State University, College of Pharmacy: Gary S. Chappell, Ph.D.

South Dakota State Medical Association: Robert D. Johnson

South Dakota Pharmaceutical Association: James Powers

Tennessee

East Tennessee State University, Quillen College of Medicine: Ernest A. Daigneault, Ph.D.

Meharry Medical College, School of Medicine: Dolores C. Shockley, Ph.D.

University of Tennessee, College of Medicine: Murray Heimberg, M.D., Ph.D.

University of Tennessee, College of Pharmacy: Dick R. Gourley, Pharm.D.

Vanderbilt University, School of Medicine: David H. Robertson, M.D.

Tennessee Pharmacists Association: Roger L. Davis, Pharm.D.

Texas

Texas A & M University, College of Medicine: Marsha A. Raebel, Pharm.D.

Texas Southern University, College of Pharmacy and Health Sciences: Eugene Hickman, Ph.D.

University of Houston, College of Pharmacy: Mustafa Lokhandwala, Ph.D.

University of Texas, Austin, College of Pharmacy: James T. Doluisio, Ph.D.

University of Texas, Medical Branch at Galveston: George T. Bryan, M.D.

University of Texas Medical School, Houston: Jacques E. Chelly, M.D., Ph.D.

University of Texas Medical School, San Antonio: Alexander M.M. Shepherd, M.D., Ph.D.

Texas Medical Association: Robert H. Barr, M.D.

Texas Pharmaceutical Association: Shirley McKee, R.Ph.

Utah

University of Utah, College of Pharmacy: David B. Roll, Ph.D.

Utah Pharmaceutical Association: Robert V. Peterson, Ph.D.

Utah Medical Association: David A. Hilding, M.D.

Vermont

University of Vermont, College of Medicine: John J. McCormack, Ph.D.

Vermont Pharmacists Association: Frederick Dobson

Virginia

Medical College of Hampton Roads: William J. Cooke, Ph.D.

Medical College of Virginia/Virginia Commonwealth Univer-

sity, School of Pharmacy: William H. Barr, Pharm.D., Ph.D.

Medical Society of Virginia: Richard W. Lindsay, M.D.

University of Virginia, School of Medicine: Peyton E. Weary, M.D.

Virginia Pharmaceutical Association: Daniel A. Herbert

Washington

Unversity of Washington, School of Pharmacy: Wendel L. Nelson, Ph.D.

Washington State University, College of Pharmacy: Martin J. Jinks, Pharm.D.

Washington State Pharmacists Association: Danial E. Baker

West Virginia

Marshall University, School of Medicine: John L. Szarek, Ph.D.

West Virginia University, School of Medicine: Douglas D. Glover, M.D.

West Virginia University Medical Center, School of Pharmacy: Arthur I. Jacknowitz, Pharm.D.

Wisconsin

Medical College of Wisconsin: Garrett J. Gross, Ph.D.

University of Wisconsin, Madison, School of Pharmacy: Chester A. Bond, Pharm.D.

University of Wisconsin Medical School, Madison: Joseph M. Benforado, M.D.

State Medical Society of Wisconsin: Thomas L. Adams, CAE

Wisconsin Pharmacists Association: Dennis Dziczkowski, R.Ph.

Wyoming

University of Wyoming, School of Pharmacy: Kenneth F. Nelson, Ph.D.

Wyoming Medical Society: R. W. Johnson, Jr.

Wyoming Pharmaceutical Association: Linda G. Sutherland

Members-at-Large

Norman W. Atwater, Ph.D., Hopewell, NJ

Cheston M. Berlin, Jr., M.D., The Milton S. Hershey Medical Center

Fred S. Brinkley, Jr., Texas State Board of Pharmacy

Herbert S. Carlin, D.Sc., Califon, NJ

Jordan Cohen, Ph.D., College of Pharmacy, University of Kentucky

John L. Cova, Ph.D., Health Insurance Association of America

Enrique Fefer, Ph.D., Pan American Health Organization

Leroy Fevang, Canadian Pharmaceutical Association

Klaus G. Florey, Ph.D., Princeton, NJ

Lester Hosto, Ph.D., Arkansas State Board of Pharmacy

Jay S. Keystone, M.D., Toronto General Hospital

Calvin M. Kunin, M.D., Ohio State University

Marvin Lipman, M.D., Scarsdale, NY

Joseph A. Mollica, Ph.D., Montcharin, DE

Stuart L. Nightingale, M.D., Food and Drug Administration

Daniel A. Nona, Ph.D., The American Council on Pharmaceutical Education

Mark Novitch, M.D., Kalamazoo, MI

Charles A. Pergola, SmithKline Beecham Consumer Brands

Donald O. Schiffman, Ph.D., Genealogy Unlimited

Carl E. Trinca, Ph.D., American Association of Colleges of Pharmacy

Members-at-Large (representing other countries that provide legal status to USP or NF)

Prof. T. D. Arias, Estafeta Universitaria, Panama, Republica de Panama

Keith Bailey, Ph.D., Canadian Bureau of Drug Research

Quintin L. Kintanar, M.D., Ph.D., Department of Health, Metro Manila, Philippines

Marcelo Jorge Vernego, Ph.D., Buenos Aires, Argentina

Members-at-Large (Public)

Clement Bezold, Ph.D., Alternative Futures Association

Alexander Grant, Food and Drug Administration

Grace Powers Monaco, J.D., Washington, DC

Paul G. Rogers, National Council on Patient Information and Education

Frances M. West, J.D., Wilmington, DE

Ex-Officio Members

Joseph M. Benforado, M.D., Madison, WI
Joseph P. Buckley, Ph.D., Houston, TX
Estelle G. Cohen, M.A., Baltimore, MD
Leo E. Hollister, M.D., Houston, TX
Paul F. Parker, D.Sc., Lexington, KY

Committee Chairmen

Credentials Committee: Peyton E. Weary, M.D.
Nominating Committee for the General Committee of Revision: Walter L. Way, M.D.
Nominating Committee for Officers and Trustees: Joseph M. Benforado, M.D.
Resolutions Committee: J. Richard Crout, M.D.
General Committee of Revision: Jerome A. Halperin
Constitution and Bylaws Committee: John V. Bergen, Ph.D.

Honorary Members

George F. Archambault, Pharm.D., J.D., Bethesda, MD
William J. Kinnard, Jr., Ph.D., Baltimore, MD
Lloyd C. Miller, Ph.D., Escondido, CA
John H. Moyer, M.D., D.Sc., Palmyra, PA
John A. Owen, Jr., M.D., Charlottesville, VA
Harry C. Shirkey, M.D., Cincinnati, OH
Linwood F. Tice, D.Sc., Philadelphia, PA

INDEX

Brand names appear in italics. Generic or family names appear in standard typeface.

A

Accupep HPF, 47
Alfacalcidol, 173
Alitraq, 47
Alka-Mints, 21
Almora, 75
Alpha tocopherol, 183
Alphamin, 167
Amin-Aid, 47
Amino-Opti-E, 183
Amitone, 21
Anacobin, 167
Apo-C, 3
Apo-Cal, 21
Apo-Ferrous Gluconate, 61
Apo-Ferrous Sulfate, 61
Apo-Folic, 55
Apo-K, 111
AquaMEPHYTON, 191

Aquasol A, 157
Aquasol E, 183
Ascorbic Acid (Vitamin C), Systemic, 3
Ascorbicap, 3
Attain, 47

B

Bedoz, 167
Beesix, 125
Beta-Carotene—for Dietary Supplement (Vitamin), Systemic, 13
Betaxin, 153
Bewon, 153
Biamine, 153
Biotin, Systemic, 19

C

Calcarb 600, 21
Calci-Chew, 21
Calciday 667, 21
Calcifediol, 173
Calciferol, 173
Calciferol Drops, 173
Calciject, 21
Calcijex, 173
Calcilac, 21
Calci-Mix, 21
Calcite 500, 21
Calcitriol, 173
Calcium 600, 21
Calcium Carbonate,
    21
Calcium Chloride, 21
Calcium Citrate, 22
Calcium Glubionate,
    22
Calcium Gluceptate &
    Calcium Gluconate,
    22
Calcium Gluconate, 22
Calcium Glucono-Ga-
    lacto Gluconate, 22
Calcium Glycerophos-
    phate & Calcium
    Lactate, 22
Calcium Lactate, 22
Calcium Lactate-Gluco-
    nate & Calcium Car-
    bonate, 22

Calcium pantothenate,
    97
Calcium-Sandoz, 21
Calcium-Sandoz Forte,
    21
Calcium Stanley, 21
Calcium Supplements,
    Systemic, 21
Calderol, 173
Calglycine, 21
Calphosan, 21
Cal-Plus, 21
Calsan, 21
Caltrate 600, 21
Caltrate Jr., 21
*Carnation Instant
    Breakfast,* 47
*Carnation Instant
    Breakfast No Sugar
    Added,* 47
Casec, 47
Cebid Timecelles, 3
Cecon, 3
Cecore 500, 3
Cee-500, 3
Cemill, 3
Cena-K, 111
Cenolate, 3
Cetane, 3
Cevi-Bid, 3
Ce-Vi-Sol, 3
Chloromag, 75
Chooz, 21
Chromic Chloride,
    37

Chromium, 37
Chromium Supplements, Systemic, 37
Citracal, 21
Citracal Liquitabs, 21
CitriSource, 47
Citroma, 75
Citro-Mag, 75
Citrotein, 47
Cobex, 167
Cobolin-M, 167
Coenzyme R, 19
Compleat Modified, 47
Compleat Regular, 47
Comply, 47
Concentrated Phillips' Milk of Magnesia, 75
Copper Gluconate, 41
Copper Supplements, Systemic, 41
Criticare HN, 47
Crystamine, 167
Crysti-12, 167
Cupric Sulfate, 41
Cupri-Pak, 41
Cyanocobalamin, 167
Cyanoject, 167
Cyomin, 167

D

DHT, 173
DHT Intensol, 173
Dibasic Calcium Phosphate, 22
Dicarbosil, 21
Dihydrotachysterol, 173
Doxine, 125
Drisdol, 173
Drisdol Drops, 173

E

E-200 I.U. Softgels, 183
E-1000 I.U. Softgels, 183
E-400 I.U. in a Water Soluble Base, 183
E-Complex-600, 183
Effer-K, 111
Elementra, 47
Endur-Acin, 91
Enercal, 48
Ensure, 47
Ensure with Fiber, 47
Ensure High Protein, 48
Ensure HN, 47
Ensure Plus, 47
Ensure Plus HN, 47

Enteral nutrition formulas, blenderized, 49

Enteral nutrition formulas, disease-specific, 49

Enteral nutrition formulas, fiber-containing, 49

Enteral nutrition formulas, milk-based, 49

Enteral nutrition formulas, modular, 49

Enteral nutrition formulas, monomeric (elemental), 49

Enteral nutrition formulas, polymeric, 49

Enteral Nutrition Formulas, Systemic, 47

Entrition Half-Strength, 47

Entrition HN, 47

Ergocalciferol, 173

E-Vitamin Succinate, 183

F

Femiron, 61
Feosol, 61

Feostat, 61
Feostat Drops, 61
Feratab, 61
Fer-Gen-Sol, 61
Fergon, 61
Fer-In-Sol Capsules, 61
Fer-In-Sol Drops, 61
Fer-In-Sol Syrup, 61
Fer-Iron Drops, 61
Fero-Grad, 61
Fero-Gradumet, 61
Ferospace, 61
Ferralet, 61
Ferralet Slow Release, 61
Ferralyn Lanacaps, 61
Ferra-TD, 61
Ferrous Fumarate, 61
Ferrous Gluconate, 61
Ferrous Sulfate, 61
Fertinic, 61
Fiberlan, 47
Fibersource, 47
Fibersource HN, 47
Flavorcee, 3
Flozenges, 139
Fluor-A-Day, 139
Fluoritab, 139
Fluoritabs, 139
Fluorodex, 139

Fluorosol, 139
Flura, 139
Flura-Drops, 139
Flura-Loz, 139
Folic Acid (Vitamin
B₉), Systemic,
55
Folvite, 55
Fumasorb, 61
Fumerin, 61

G

Gencalc 600, 21
Gen-K, 111
Glucerna, 47
Glu-K, 111
Gramcal, 21
Great Shake, 47

H

Hemocyte, 61
Hepatic-Aid II, 47
Hydrobexan, 167
Hydro-Cobex, 167
Hydro-Crysti-12,
167
Hydroxocobalamin,
167
Hydroxy-Cobal, 167

Hytakerol, 173
Hytinic, 61

I

Immun-Aid, 47
Impact, 47
Impact with Fiber, 47
InFeD, 61
Introlan, 47
Introlite, 47
Iodopen, 147
Ircon, 61
Iron Dextran, 61
Iron-Polysaccharide, 61
Iron Sorbitol, 61
Iron Supplements, Sys-
temic, 61
Isocal, 47
Isocal HCN, 47
Isocal HN, 47
Isolan, 47
Isosource, 47
Isosource HN, 47
Isotein HN, 47

J

Jectofer, 61
Jevity, 47

K

K-8, 111
K-10, 111
Kalcinate, 21
Kalium Durules, 111
Kaochlor-10, 111
Kaochlor-20, 111
Kaochlor 10%, 111
Kaochlor S-F 10%, 111
Kaon, 111
Kaon-Cl, 111
Kaon-Cl-10, 111
Kaon-Cl 20% Liquid, 111
Karidium, 139
Kato, 111
Kay Ciel, 111
Kaylixir, 111
KCL 5%, 111
K-Dur, 111
K-Electrolyte, 111
K-G Elixir, 111
K-Ide, 111
K-Lease, 111
K-Long, 111
K-Lor, 111
Klor-Con 8, 111
Klor-Con 10, 111
Klor-Con/EF, 111
Klor-Con Powder, 111
Klor-Con/25 Powder, 111
Klorvess, 111

Klorvess Effervescent Granules, 111
Klorvess 10% Liquid, 111
Klotrix, 111
K-Lyte, 111
K-Lyte/Cl, 111
K-Lyte/Cl 50, 111
K-Lyte/Cl Powder, 111
K-Lyte DS, 111
K-Med 900, 111
K-Norm, 111
Kolyum, 111
Konakion, 191
K-Phos M. F., 101
K-Phos Neutral, 101
K-Phos No. 2, 101
K-Phos Original, 101
K+ 10, 111
K+ Care, 111
K+ Care ET, 111
K-Sol, 111
K-Tab, 111
K-Vescent, 111

L

LA-12, 167
Lipisorb; 47
Liquid-Cal, 21
Liquid Cal-600, 21
Liqui-E, 183

Lonalac, 47
Luride, 139
Luride Lozi-Tabs, 139
Luride-SF Lozi-Tabs, 139

M

Maalox Antacid Caplets, 21
Mag 2, 75
Mag-200, 75
Mag-L-100, 75
Maglucate, 75
Magnacal, 47
Magnesium Chloride, 75
Magnesium Citrate, 75
Magnesium Glucep-tate, 75
Magnesium glucohep-tonate, 75
Magnesium Gluco-nate, 75
Magnesium Hydrox-ide, 75
Magnesium Lactate, 75
Magnesium Oxide, 75
Magnesium Pidolate, 75
Magnesium pyrogluta-mate, 75
Magnesium-Rougier, 75
Magnesium Sulfate, 75
Magnesium Supple-ments, Systemic, 75
Magonate, 75
Mag-Ox 400, 75
Mag-Tab SR, 75
Magtrate, 75
Mallamint, 21
Manganese Chloride, 83
Manganese Sulfate, 83
Manganese Supple-ments, Systemic, 83
Maox, 75
Max-Caro, 13
MCT Oil, 47
Mega-C/A Plus, 3
Menadiol, 191
Menu Magic Instant Breakfast, 47
Menu Magic Milk Shake, 47
Mephyton, 191
Meritene, 47
MGP, 75
Micro-K, 111
Micro-K 10, 111
Micro-K LS, 111
Microlipid, 47
Moducal, 47

Mol-Iron, 61
Molybdenum Supplements, Systemic, 87
Molypen, 87

N

Neo-Calglucon, 21
Neo-Fer, 61
Neo-K, 111
Nephro-Calci, 21
Nephro-Fer, 61
Nepro, 47
Nestrex, 125
Neuroforte-R, 167
Neutra-Phos, 101
Neutra-Phos-K, 101
Nia-Bid, 91
Niac, 91
Niacels, 91
Niacin, 91
Niacin (Vitamin B$_3$), Systemic, 91
Niacinamide, 91
Niacor, 91
Nico-400, 91
Nicobid Tempules, 91
Nicolar, 91
Nicotinamide, 91
Nicotinex Elixir, 91
Nicotinic acid, 91
Niferex, 61

Niferex-150, 61
Novoferrogluc, 61
Novoferrosulfa, 61
Novo-Folacid, 55
Novofumar, 61
Novo-Niacin, 91
Nu-Cal, 21
Nu-Iron, 61
Nu-Iron 150, 61
Nutren 1.0, 47
Nutren 1.0 with Fiber, 47
Nutren 1.5, 47
Nutren 2.0, 47
NutriHep, 47
Nutrilan Flavored Supplements, 47
NutriSource, 47
NutriSource HN, 47
NutriVent, 47

O

One-Alpha, 173
Orazinc, 197
Ortho/CS, 3
Os-Cal, 21
Os-Cal Chewable, 21
Os-Cal 500, 21
Os-Cal 500 Chewable, 21
Osmolite, 47
Osmolite HN, 47

Ostoforte, 173
Oysco, 21
Oysco 500 Chewable, 21
Oyst-Cal 500, 21
Oystercal 500, 21

P

Palafer, 61
Pantothenic Acid (Vitamin B$_5$), Systemic, 97
PDF, 139
Pediaflor, 139
Pediasure, 47
Pediasure with Fiber, 47
Pedi-Dent, 139
Peptamen, 47
Perative, 48
Pharmaflur, 139
Pharmaflur 1.1, 139
Pharmaflur df, 139
Pheryl-E, 183
Phillips' Chewable Tablets, 75
Phillips' Magnesia Tablets, 75
Phillips' Milk of Magnesia, 75
Phillips' Milk of Mag-

nesia, Concentrated, 75
Phos-Flur, 139
Phosphates, Systemic, 101
Phytomenadione, 191
Phytonadione, 191
PMS Egozinc, 197
PMS Ferrous Sulfate, 61
Polycose, 48
Posture, 21
Potasalan, 111
Potassium Acetate, 112
Potassium Bicarbonate, 112
Potassium Bicarbonate & Potassium Chloride, 112
Potassium Bicarbonate & Potassium Citrate, 112
Potassium Chloride, 112
Potassium Gluconate, 112
Potassium Gluconate & Potassium Chloride, 112
Potassium Gluconate & Potassium Citrate, 112

Potassium Phosphates, 101
Potassium-Rougier, 112
Potassium-Sandoz, 112
Potassium & Sodium Phosphates, 101
Potassium Supplements, Systemic, 111
Potassium triplex, 112
Pre-Attain, 48
Precision HN, 48
Precision Isotonic Diet, 48
Precision Low Residue, 48
Primabalt, 167
Profiber, 48
ProMod, 48
Promote, 48
Propac, 48
Protain XL, 48
Provatene, 13
Pulmocare, 48
Pyri, 125
Pyridoxine (Vitamin B$_6$), Systemic, 125

R

Radiostol Forte, 173
Reabilan, 48

Reabilan HN, 48
Replete, 48
Replete with Fiber, 48
Resource, 48
Resource Plus, 48
Retinol, 157
Riboflavin (Vitamin B$_2$), Systemic, 131
Rocaltrol, 173
Rodex, 125
Rolaids Calcium Rich, 21
Roychlor-10%, 112
Rubesol-1000, 167
Rubramin PC, 167
Rum-K, 111

S

Selenious Acid, 135
Selenium, 135
Selenium Supplements, Systemic, 135
Sele-Pak, 135
Selepen, 135
Shovite, 167
Simron, 61
Slo-Niacin, 91
Slow Fe, 61
Slow-K, 111
Slow-Mag, 75

Sodium Fluoride, Systemic, 139
Sodium Iodide, Systemic, 147
Sodium Phosphates, 101
Solatene, 13
Solu-Flur, 139
Span-FF, 61
Stresstein, 48
Sumacal, 48
Sunkist, 3
Suplena, 48
Sustacal, 48
Sustacal 8.8, 48
Sustacal with Fiber, 48
Sustacal HC, 48
Sustagen, 48
Synkayvite, 191

T

Tasty Shake, 48
Ten-K, 111
Thiamine (Vitamin B₁), Systemic, 153
Titralac, 21
Tolerex, 48
TraumaCal, 48
Traum-Aid HBC, 48
Travasorb Hepatic Diet, 48

Travasorb HN, 48
Travasorb Renal Diet, 48
Travasorb STD, 48
Tribasic Calcium Phosphate, 22
Tri-K, 111
Trikates, 112
Tums, 21
Tums 500, 21
Tums E-X, 21
Tums Extra Strength, 21
Tums Regular Strength, 21
Twin-K, 111
TwoCal HN, 48

U

Ultracal, 48
Ultralan, 48
Uro-KP-Neutral, *101*
Uro-Mag, 75

V

Verazinc, 197
Vibal, 167
Vibal LA, 167
Vita Plus E, 183

Vitabee 6, 167
Vitabee 12, 125
Vital High Nitrogen,
   48
Vitamin A, Systemic,
   157
Vitamin B₃, 91
Vitamin B₅, 97
Vitamin B₉, 55
Vitamin B₁₂, Sys-
   temic, 167
Vitamin Bw, 19
Vitamin C, 3
Vitamin D & Related
   Compounds,
   Systemic, 173
Vitamin E, Systemic,
   183
Vitamin H, 19
Vitamin K, Systemic,
   191
Vitaneed, 48

Vivonex T.E.N.,
   48

W

Webber Vitamin E, 183

Z

Zinc 15, 197
Zinc-220, 197
Zinc Chloride, 197
Zinc Gluconate, 197
Zinc Sulfate, 197
Zinc Supplements,
   Systemic, 197
Zinca-Pak, 197
Zincate, 197

Expertly detailed, pharmaceutical guides
can now be at your fingertips
from U.S. Pharmacopeia

THE USP GUIDE TO MEDICINES
78092-5/$6.99 US/$8.99 Can

- More than 2,000 entries for both prescription
  and non-prescription drugs
- Handsomely detailed color insert

THE USP GUIDE
TO HEART MEDICINES
78094-1/$6.99 US/$8.99 Can

- Side effects and proper dosages for over 400
  brand-name and generic drugs
- Breakdown of heart ailments such as angina,
  high cholesterol and high blood pressure

THE USP GUIDE TO
VITAMINS AND MINERALS
78093-3/$6.99 US/$8.99 Can

- Precautions for children, senior citizens and
  pregnant women
- Latest findings and benefits of dietary supplements